AN ANTHROPOLOGY OF LYING:
INFORMATION IN THE
DOCTOR–PATIENT RELATIONSHIP

An Anthropology of Lying: Information in the Doctor–Patient Relationship

SYLVIE FAINZANG

National Institute for Health and Medical Research (INSERM), France

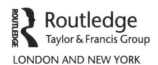

Routledge
Taylor & Francis Group

LONDON AND NEW YORK

First published 2015 by Ashgate Publishing

Published 2016 by Routledge
2 Park Square, Milton Park, Abingdon, Oxfordshire OX14 4RN
711 Third Avenue, New York, NY 10017, USA

First issued in paperback 2016

Routledge is an imprint of the Taylor & Francis Group, an informa business

This book was first published in French by the Presses Universitaires de France in 2006, under the title: *La relation médecins-malades: information et mensonge*. It has been translated from French by Jenefer Bonczyk.

British Library Cataloguing in Publication Data
A catalogue record for this book is available from the British Library.

The Library of Congress has cataloged the printed edition as follows:
Fainzang, Sylvie, 1954– , author.
  An anthropology of lying : information in the doctor–patient relationship / by Sylvie Fainzang.
     p. ; cm.
  Includes bibliographical references and index.
  ISBN 978-1-4724-5602-1 (hardback)
  I. Title.
  [DNLM: 1. Physician–Patient Relations. 2. Truth Disclosure. 3. Deception. 4. Ethics,
Professional. 5. Patient Rights. W 62]
  R727.3
  610.69'6—dc23

                                                                      2014037347

ISBN 13: 978-1-138-70214-1 (pbk)
ISBN 13: 978-1-4724-5602-1 (hbk)

Contents

Contents

Introduction

The Cretan philosopher Epimenides says: 'All Cretans are liars'. If he is telling the truth then he is himself a liar since he is Cretan. Therefore he is not telling the truth. And so he is himself a liar. Therefore he is telling the truth. Consequently, Cretans are not liars at all. And so it follows that Epimenides is not a liar either. Therefore he lied …

('The liar paradox', imagined by Euclid)

It is pertinent today to take an interest in the issue of information — since our times are characterised by its glorification, and show signs of becoming information-obsessed. This issue is also frequently discussed within the framework of the doctor–patient relationship. However, it is less common to investigate the true nature of this information and its links with truth in particular. But it is more problematic, even totally irreverential, to tackle a subject such as lying and consider it as a social phenomenon, especially when choosing to examine both the lies doctors tell patients and those patients tell doctors, insisting on studying them in the same anthropological terms. Lying is however common practice within this relationship even though each protagonist should be conveying information to the other in order to obtain optimal care. And so, what is the place of lying within the doctor–patient relationship and within information exchanges between actors? What is the nature of the information patients receive concerning their illness, and what is the nature of the information they hope for? How is this quest for information carried out in the context of the doctor–patient relationship, and how is the information conveyed? How do patients perceive this information and the way in which it is given in the context of their relationship with the doctors? What role does information play in their therapeutic choices? Such are the questions guiding this research conducted in France, based on observation of the disparity, or even the contradiction, between the discourse of patients who complain they are not being informed about their condition, and the discourse of doctors who claim that patients do not want to know of their true condition. The twin aims of this research are to expose the conditions in which patients are informed and to understand what is being played out inside the doctor–patient relationship in terms of patient information. In other words, the objective is to gauge both the perception and the reality of the relationships individuals maintain with medical authority. The information in question partly concerns how the diagnosis, or the prognosis, is conveyed, but it also relates to the effects, risks and benefits of treatments. It will thus be examined on these multiple levels.

The information that patients receive concerning their affliction and their treatment is one of the central issues in the debate surrounding the position of patients in the healthcare system and in the therapeutic relationship. But this question is generally asked in ethical terms and many works take it as their object precisely in order to defend a certain position. The authors discussing patient information tend to highlight the ethical questions raised by formulating a prognosis or by asking patients to give consent when they do not possess sufficient information to make their decision. This however is not the aim of this work. Here, the perspective is that of the social sciences. In other words, the purpose is to analyse situations without inferring a normative position.

The issue of information revolves primarily around that of truth. Medical literature abounds with commentaries on the theme of truth which investigate the question of how to decide whether to tell the patient the truth or not. Some authors have shown that for certain pathologies such as cancer (for example Saillant 1988), the problem goes beyond the question of whether or not to tell the truth because there is great uncertainty in knowledge in the domain. However, as we will see, although this uncertainty is indeed an obstacle to truth and, above all, an argument for doctors to justify denying their patients the truth, this is only one aspect of the much bigger issue of information provision. Thus, the issue of truth should be examined in a comprehensive but also extensive manner. The notion of truth, for which Fletcher (1979) distinguished between logical truth (accuracy) and moral truth (veracity), is clearly connected to the notion of lying. According to Fletcher, logical truth is the correspondence between verbal expression and the problem to which this expression refers, whereas moral truth is the correspondence between the expression given to our thought and the thought itself. Logical truth is thus the truth as we know it:[1] moral truth is the truth corresponding to what we believe to be true. Here, it is the second meaning that interests us: that which the liar believes to be true.

The use of the term 'lie' in this work is deliberate, since it does not only apply to a truth not told or to so-called 'lying by omission', but to the possible communication of false information. Simmel (1991) showed that social relationships involve a certain degree of reciprocal dissimulation. In his view, what distinguishes a lie is not that the person being duped has a false idea of reality – since this is something that a lie shares with a mistake – but that the person being lied to is misled about the liar's opinion.

The aim of this study is not to add yet another opinion to the numerous views expressed on the question of whether or not it is better for the patient

---

1   In other words, that which derives from knowledge. On this subject Dausset wrote: 'one day's truths can be discredited the next' (cited by Maurice Olender, 1983).

to be told the truth, but instead, to identify the arguments protagonists in the doctor–patient relationship use to explain their behaviour, and above all, to understand what their positions and practices conceal and imply. In this way, I will attempt to define the cognitive and moral systems with which the actors' positions are associated, and to assess how well practices comply with discourses in order to understand in concrete terms how information is used, sought, disclosed and withheld. Thus, this study does not seek to lend support to a certain point of view by showing the benefit or harm that knowing the truth can have on a patient's health or morale, nor does it seek to make any judgement on the practices studied. Many doctors have given their personal thoughts on this subject and the validity of their reflections will not be called into question here. The aim is to attempt to understand what the doctors on one side, and the patients on the other, say to justify their actions and to analyse this behaviour without passing judgement, in a relationship of 'anthropological empathy' towards the two parties. This is done without endorsing the discourse of one over the other since both discourses are considered to be equally valid, each with their own reasons and logics. Additionally, because I was examining the issue of information within the framework of the doctor–patient relationship, I also chose to investigate the information provided by patients.[2]

This approach supposed a certain number of epistemological conditions. Firstly, it involved taking as a starting point what the subject believes to be true, in other words, to start, from an emic point of view, from what the author of the lie believes to be the truth. Next, it supposed the acceptance of the iconoclastic nature of the term 'lie' as applied to the medical profession. Indeed, the practice of lying is present within this professional milieu even though practitioners would generally object to calling it that because it is rationalised and even legitimised in this context. But is it not the role of the social sciences to burn the icons when necessary?

One path I was inclined to take at the beginning of my research was that of any legal action taken by patients, not to study the phenomenon in its legal phase, but to determine on what grounds, and at what point, patient resentment at not being informed is transformed into a public and legal complaint. Although various authors have taken an interest in patient associations and have concluded that more and more patients are taking the initiative and becoming actors in the care of their health problems and the management of their therapy (Rabeharisoa and Callon 1999), my inquiries however did not lead me down this

---

2 Of course, it is impossible to completely separate information from lying or to study doctors on one side and patients on the other, since the analysis takes place wholly within this relationship. The structure of this work simply serves as a convenient means of presenting the materials gathered concerning the representations and practices of both parties, of which I will endeavour to present all the linkages and ramifications.

path. In truth, such recourse to justice is not in any way the most common behaviour within the patient population. Besides, to use the simple existence of patient associations as a means of inferring the behaviour of the 'contemporary patient' would be to take a biased view of the issue. Certainly, the existence of these associations reveals an increased willingness to act against the paternalistic model, and the fact that these Patient Associations have been federated in France into the 'Inter-associations Group on Healthcare' (a collective of associations representing families, consumers, patients and disabled people) shows their desire to build an opposing force to medical power by setting up an institutional role for the user and by facilitating direct participation. However, for one thing, the type of people who join these associations are not particularly representative of all patients,[3] and for another, one can belong to an association whose head office is making certain demands without necessarily sharing the same attitudes oneself.[4]

In fact, many patients complain about a situation but never actually take legal action. This allows us to assess the plural dimension of the notion of complaint. As it happened, among all the patients I met, while a certain number expressed real dissatisfaction, none had transformed their confidential complaint into a legal complaint; in other words, none had turned their dissatisfaction into denunciation.

Lying between doctors and patients − which should be approached as a practice that both parties partake in − is complicated by the fact that it is marred by judgements, which diverge according to *who* is lying and in what context. Although this study makes no moral judgement on the issue, it does however attempt to examine the mechanisms that come into play when society and the protagonists themselves make differing judgements. The various ways in which a doctor's lie is justified or put into perspective do not stop it from being a lie, but these justifications are in themselves prime examples of the social place a doctor's lie holds within the therapeutic relationship. Indeed, a lie is given a different value depending on how the author or the recipient of

---

3   The existence of associations in itself does not appear to me to be sufficient to describe the behaviour of contemporary patients, if only because the most powerful associations are those fighting against AIDS, and in all western countries, these associations grew out of the homosexual movement (see Broca 2003) which established a particular link with global society and criticism of the current health system.

4   The massive campaign aiming to expand patient powers and strengthen their right to information was largely driven by the specific circumstances created by AIDS. While this had some impact on the doctor–patient relationship in general, it is not however sure that it gave rise to models of relationships which are identical for other pathologies. Even though there are many patient associations today (in the fields of muscular dystrophy, cancer and many others) and meetings have been organised between AIDS campaigners and the *Ligue contre le cancer* (League Against Cancer) (Dodier 2002), not all patients belong to associations, far from it.

the lie is regarded, the role each of these actors play in social relationships (including medical relationships) and the personal or social reasons that structure it. Evidently, whether a lie is to be valued or condemned is linked to the social context within which it is told. The value given to a lie changes since it is generally considered to be positive when told by a doctor, and negative when told by a patient. A doctor's lie is deemed to be acceptable, but a patient's is not. Within the medical relationship, a lie is thus not perceived in the same way depending on who says it and the position they occupy.

We should not consider doctors and patients to be necessarily antagonistic, and to be in a relationship where the former are always trying to keep the information to themselves and the latter are forever trying to obtain it. The profiles are more diversified than that and the situation is much less dualistic. I will try to fairly represent this diversity while highlighting the key features which distinguish the groups of actors, partly based on the structural character of the doctor–patient relationship.

Finally, in contrast to some studies carried out in the field of public health (see for example Demma et al. 1999), this study does not aim to define the needs and expectations of patients. As such, no recommendations are made here: each reader will want to draw different conclusions, these could be technical for some (those looking for elements likely to improve the conditions of patient information) and sociological for others (those searching for elements that shed light on the mechanisms that govern the doctor–patient relationship as a social relationship). This work thus intends to take the first steps in an anthropology of lying that is free from moral expectations, not because these are not valuable but because they obscure true sociological thinking on this social phenomenon and the mechanisms behind it.

The Law and Legal Texts

The principle of information is defined in numerous legislative texts and charters such as the *Code de déontologie médicale* (Code of Medical Ethics), the *Code de la santé publique* (Code of Public Health) and recommendations by ANAES (French National Health Evaluation and Accreditation Agency). For example, article L.1111-2 of the Code of Public Health, reformed by the Act of 4 March 2002, stipulates that everyone has the right to be informed on the state of their health. This information is of upmost importance and Article L. 1111-4 specifies that 'everyone takes decisions concerning their health with the help of a health professional and the information and recommendations they provide'. In truth, legislative texts that guarantee patient rights were put in place before this law was enacted, and among these rights was that of information. Numerous texts and professional codes on patient rights exist, on a national level in France (Huriet's Law, 1988; Bioethical Laws, 1994; the New Code of Medical Ethics, 1995; the updated Charter for Hospitalized Patients, 1995) and on an international level (Declaration on the Promotion of Patients' Rights in Europe by the WHO, for example[5]), see Khodoss (2000).

Article 35 of the Code of Medical Ethics (of 6 September 1995) envisages that: 'Doctors owe the person they examine care, advice and information that is loyal, clear and appropriate to his/her condition and the examinations and care proposed. For the duration of the illness, the doctor must take the patients' personality into account when providing explanations and be aware of their level of understanding'. For their part, the ANAES recommendations aimed at doctors stated in 2000 that 'patient information should comprise explanations on the illness and its development, diagnostic and therapeutic steps, adverse side-effects and potential risks, even the most improbable', recommendations re-iterated today in the 'Plan Cancer' (Cancer Action Plan).

Incidentally, all European health systems today are moving towards an increased respect for patients' individual rights. This phenomenon has been accelerated in France by several health scandals which prompted deeper questioning of doctors. These scandals have greatly eroded patient confidence in doctors and led to what has been called a crisis of legitimacy in medicine (Aïach et al. 1994; Dodier 2002). It has also been helped by the *Etats Généraux de la Santé* (French Health Conference) in 1998, during which patient associations reiterated their demands, and in particular, their desire to have access to genuine information. E. Caniard (2001) thus emphasises the link between the Health Conference and the law on Patient Rights and Quality in the Healthcare System.

This important event gave rise to, firstly, an announcement by the prime minister of measures aimed at allowing patients direct access to their medical files, and secondly, to numerous publications on today's revolution in the status of patients in our healthcare system and in the doctor–patient relationship. For example, Gillot (2000) wrote that today 'being ill no longer involves resignedly giving up ones rights and prerogatives', but that 'on the contrary, it involves affirming one's position as a user of the health system and asserting one's rights as regards this position', and that 'this is a case of a large-scale mutation in social relationships'.

In other societies as well as in other health-care systems, authors discussing the doctor–patient relationship generally agree that a radical change is occurring in its paradigm. Charles et al. (1999) thus identified three principal models

---

5   The WHO Declaration on the Promotion of Patients' Rights in Europe, 1994, thus stipulates in Art. 2 that: 'Patients have the right to be fully informed about their health status, including the medical facts about their condition, about the proposed medical procedures, together with the potential risks and benefits of each procedure, and about alternatives to the proposed procedures'.

(the paternalistic model, the model of shared decision-making, and the model of informed decision-making). The paternalistic approach is based on the idea that doctors know what is best for their patients. This legitimisation of medical control was supported by ethical codes urging doctors to act 'in the best interests of patients'. This led the different actors to expect doctors to play a dominant role in the decision-making process. In the 1980s, questions started to be asked as to the credibility of this assertion and the models of shared and informed decision-making were developed, largely, they explain, in reaction to the paternalistic model.

However, when examining the facts, several authors have expressed their doubts as to whether, in France at least, such a modification in the doctor–patient relationship has really occurred. They believe that patients are still not really informed, particularly in the context of hospital medicine. As such, although numerous declarations exist that stress the need for patient information – based either on the ethical and political presupposition that informing citizens is essential for the democratic process to function and contributes to the promotion of respect for citizen autonomy and dignity, or on pragmatic considerations, since informing patients contributes to improvements in the quality of care – Ghadi (2001), for instance, believes that, in a large number of cases, producing written documents for the patient to sign is aimed more at protecting doctors from legal consequences if one of the treatments' potential risks occurs, than clearly informing the patient. Even though the 1994 Declaration on the Promotion of Patients' Rights in Europe specifies one's right as a patient to be fully informed of one's health status, and of the risks and advantages of the medical acts proposed, and even though in response to patient associations' requests for access to medical documents without medical intermediaries the public authorities have promised patients this direct access to their own files, the reality today is nowhere near this ideal and the patient's file is still often only communicated to the GPs. Ponchon's (1998) observation that in reality it is the GP's information that is sought after, with the idea that the patient is incapable of understanding the contents of the document, is still valid today.

It appears in fact, from reading all these works, that the way patients are informed today, as practiced by the professionals and recommended by the texts, is more in answer to judicial concerns than for ethical or therapeutic reasons, and it is very often through a fear of prosecution that the doctors choose to inform their patients. The legislation was written in response to the demands of the patient associations, but it does not reflect a shared desire of the whole medical community to enable patients to gain access to information concerning their illnesses and their bodies, even though some medical staff willingly agree with providing information for therapeutic reasons. The model of shared decision-making itself appears to have been created more out of a fear of prosecution than through the doctors' convictions, some of whom prove to be very reluctant, unless it is strictly specified by the law, to provide patients with information on the state of their body and their care. It is as if Hippocrates' recommendations remain valid,[6] though, according to Lagrée (2002): 'Sitting between the paternalism of Hippocrates widely practiced by the medical body until a recent date, and information at all costs and without precaution dear to North Americans today, a good deal of thinking has led us, from the Nuremberg Code to the jurisprudence of the beginning of the 21st century, to insist more and more on enlightened consent on the part of the patient'. Informed consent appears to be only very partially required. Broclain (2001) cites, for example, the lack of requests for consent for routine examinations in a cardiology ward and believes that there is still a long way to go before the autonomist paradigm becomes common practice.[7] The gap that exists between the texts of law and reality in practice is borne out on various levels and although the Public Health Code states that 'every person should have full access to all the information concerning their health detained by professionals and health institutions', close observation of the facts reveals that information often continues to be withheld from patients.[8]

However, in relation to the current legislation, the prevailing wisdom that patients are now completely informed is becoming widespread. It appears to be accepted that patients have gone from being objects to subjects,[9] and that their relationships with their doctors are of a contractual nature, in virtue of which doctors and patients share the responsibility and decision-making of therapeutic choices, thus proving their autonomy. While the legal texts show an interesting evolution in society, it is not however possible to use them as the only source when assessing the reality of this evolution.

This consensus is echoed in the abundant medical literature on the subject of patient information. These texts discuss the specific situation of contemporary patients who can choose, negotiate with the medical profession, act as informed patients and decide on the most rational health behaviours. They celebrate the

---

6   'One should do everything calmly, skilfully, concealing almost everything from the patient during the procedure, cheerfully and serenely giving appropriate encouragement … without letting the patient be aware of anything that may occur or of the threat he faces: since more than one patient has been caused much distress by a prognosis where he was told of what could happen to him or the threat he faced'. Hippocrate, in *De la bienséance*, 16, cited in Lagrée (2002).

7   In some typologies, the autonomist model has replaced the paternalist model; in this model patients have the right, as free and responsible adult citizens, to refuse to give consent to their doctors' decision, and to take on, subject to appropriate information, the role of ultimate decision-maker in care concerning them (Broclain 2001).

8   In the case of screening for breast cancer, practiced in screening centres for example, the patient is required to designate a doctor to receive their results rather than receiving them directly.

9   M. Reich (2004) talks of the transition from an object of rights to a subject of rights.

arrival of an era of patient autonomy, of patients who are now 'enlightened'. Indeed, the notion of 'health democracy' is underpinned by this autonomy and patient information. This notion implies a redistribution of power in the field of health in the direction of civil society (Dodier 2002; Barbot 2002; Rabeharisoa and Callon 1999) and to users in particular.

Yet, we should note that while the Code of Medical Ethics safeguards information, this is not without reservations. It stipulates that: 'Nevertheless, in the *interests* of the patient and for *legitimate* reasons assessed *in conscience* by the practitioner, a patient can be kept in *ignorance* of a *serious* diagnosis or prognosis, except in a case where his/her affliction exposes third parties to the risk of contamination' [my italics]. In the same spirit, the 1994 WHO Declaration on the Promotion of Patients' Rights in Europe envisages that 'information can only exceptionally be *withheld from patients* when there are *good reasons to believe* that it would cause them serious harm'. As we can see, the principle of information is subject to some transgressions, envisaged by the law itself. The possibility (envisaged by the law) of not informing patients and the judgement on which this is based relies on the degree of certainty on the part of the doctor, the personality of the patient and the risk of distress or despair, even if this aspect is not included, or in any case not in the same terms, in the law of 4 March 2002.

Therefore, we should question the extent to which this 'large-scale mutation in social relationships' has taken place. Do patients really possess the decision-making powers we believe them to have nowadays? In response to what appears to be a genuine revolution, we must question the nature of the social roles and the extent to which they have been reconfigured, including the nature of this autonomy, whether patients are capable of assuming this role, and whether doctors are able to let them. And consequently, what about this information? If, in the strictly legal sense, the law of 4 March 2002 (also called the Patients' Rights Act) has restricted doctor's liberty to withhold information when they deem appropriate, this information is not in fact always provided, mainly in situations where it is deemed potentially harmful to the patient — in line with the Code of Medical Ethics — and because, in the interests of patients, doctors believe that some things should not be said. One of the questions raised is thus how doctors decide what is in patients' interests, and on what basis they determine what they can and cannot say, and to whom.

This brings us to the heart of our investigation, where we reconsider the reality of information provision within the doctor–patient relationship as a prerequisite to exercising 'patient power'. The analysis leads me to demonstrate that the practices of both doctors and patients are set in social and cultural patterns which heavily restrict their actions, and to question the quasi-consensual assumption that patients are now truly enlightened.

A New Perspective

I will thus look at the issue of information primarily in terms of its links with truth and lies. This work intends to break away from the majority of studies carried out on the issue of truth in medicine – from testimonies of health-care professionals describing their own practice in order to form an ethical position on the issue, to texts written by those acting as spokespeople for patients.[10] While this work does not take an ethical stance, I will nevertheless examine the social stakes engendered by the ethical debate. This works attempts to change the perspective with which these questions are generally approached. In this respect, as a counterpoint to the psychological perspective with which the existing literature perceives the practice of lying, I intend to 'de-psychologise' the approach to the phenomenon and examine the social mechanisms at play.

The treatment of cancer provides an ideal framework for the study of these issues. A large part of the observations reproduced in this work took place in this field because this pathology remains emblematic of 'serious disease', the context in which the issue of truth tends to be discussed. However, I deliberately chose not to limit my observations to cancer pathologies because the problem of information and lying also applies in other situations, especially those associated with the concept of seriousness – even though, as we will see, this notion is itself also the object of hugely variable judgements – since the seriousness of the affliction holds a fundamental importance in the practice of information sharing or lying.

The research was carried out in the cancer and internal medicine departments of various hospitals. However, since questions concerning information and truth cannot be asked in the same way depending on the type of illness and the degree of seriousness, it was necessary to observe a wide range of situations within discrete pathological areas. The research included some 80 patients, of whom 60 had cancer (stomach, oesophagus, colon, liver, pancreas, lung, brain, breast, bladder and bone). Most had cancers of the digestive system (pancreas, colon and liver), lung and breast – a result of the specialisations within the hospital departments in which the study took place. Of all the subjects studied, 20 suffered from other pathologies such as chronic inflammatory diseases and/or auto-immune diseases (arthritis of the hip, lupus, polyarthritis, sarcoidosis, tuberculosis, scerloderma, osteoporosis, sideroblastic anaemia, unruptured aneurysms, stenosis, phlebothrombosis, Hodgkin's disease, liver damage, inflammation of the arteries, renal infarction, acute renal insufficiency, tonsillar lymphoma, and Behçet's disease).

---

10 This also applies to the book by Joseph-Jeanneney et al. (2002) (which consists of a joint reflection by the wife of a cancer patient, an oncologist and a psychologist who discuss their questions, doubts and certainties surrounding the disease: Should the whole truth be told? Should one talk differently to the family and the patient?), and also to Bataille's (2003) work.

The patients were seen at various stages of their diseases. Some were considered to be almost fully recovered and were only going to the hospital for follow-up appointments, others were undergoing treatment (chemotherapy, radiotherapy, operations), while others again were in palliative care. The patients studied were of differing ages (from 30 to 80 years old, with the majority between 55 and 70), of both sexes, and from varying socioprofessional backgrounds (secretaries, accountants, teachers, medical staff, researcher, cleaners, business leaders, soldier, shopkeepers, engineers, computer specialists, wine makers, employees, sommelier, salesperson, unemployed, administrative officers, service officers, petroleum engineer, artists, craftsmen, manual labourers, no profession). The patients who took part in the study did not however make up a sample in the strict sense of the term, which would have involved faithfully representing the general population in terms of age group, sex and socioprofessional background. Nevertheless, the group of informants was sufficiently diversified to enable me to unearth consistencies within the social, cultural and demographic categories concerned. As is common in qualitative research, the group of informants was formed during the research process in the hospitals visited. An inquiry aiming to set up a representative sample would need to make an *a priori* selection of the people to be studied and so go against the anthropological method which is based on immersion and empathy.

On a practical level, I had the opportunity to be present during consultations and observe the process. I then met the doctors and patients separately. Additionally, I met some patients again and others for the first time during visits to the hospital wards. My aim was to multiply and diversify the contexts in which patients were interviewed in order to obtain different kinds of material and broaden the scope of the data. The aim was to highlight certain logics and mechanisms underlying the exchanges between doctors and patients. The places of study will not be specified here since my intention is not to write a monograph, and as such, identifying the hospital departments and the actors involved would add nothing useful to the conclusions of the study. On the contrary, my position is to scrupulously respect people's anonymity, and the initials, that will sometimes appear simply to render the presentation of the material more alive, have all been changed. This study is based on materials gathered in various different ways. I used open-ended interviews with patients to collect accounts of illness and therapeutic journeys, paying attention to the context in which the illness appeared, the different steps of the care they received, the questions they asked themselves and those they did and did not ask the medical staff, the answers they received, the conditions in which they were told their diagnosis, the information they received or did not receive and their subsequent reactions. I also carried out unstructured interviews with 12 doctors, which consisted of defining how the doctors viewed the issue of information and perceived patient expectations, in order to measure the potential gap between the stated aspirations of the patients and those the doctors believe them to hold. Finally, as a fundamental element of the inquiry, the observation of consultations helped me to study the manner in which verbal exchanges between doctors and patients take place in this context.

When possible, I questioned the doctors and patients directly after the consultation I had observed. Otherwise, I met them again later, sometimes several days after the event. For some, these interviews took the form of a sort of 'debriefing', in which they explained what they had said, and why they had said it, what they had not said and why they had not. To do this, I met the subjects both at the hospital (in different contexts: consultation rooms, outpatient departments, during week-long hospital stays and at meetings of healthcare personnel), but also away from the hospital environment, notably at the patient's homes where they tended to talk more freely. This was done in order to diversify the spaces of interaction with the informants, whether they were patients, doctors, other healthcare workers or the patient's family. The interviews at the patient's homes either took place at my proposal or at their unsolicited invitation. Others telephoned or emailed to inform me of a development in their treatment or in their relationship with their doctor.

I had wanted to follow the patients in any support groups or advocacy groups they might participate in, in order to see if and how patients sought information there or voiced their grievances concerning a lack thereof. However, none of the patients studied went down this route. In fact, many patients refuse to join support groups and patient associations to avoid what they consider to be a morbid atmosphere. Although this research reveals that many patients feel they are insufficiently informed, very few of them seek to formalise their grievances or express them within established groups. Given this, I went to the spaces that patients regularly frequent, namely, consulting rooms and inpatient services.

Interviewing patients and doctors in parallel allowed me to better understand the actions, words and reactions of each actor within the doctor–patient relationship, and to better appreciate their reasons and the mechanisms at play. The inevitable empathy that develops between researcher and subject in an anthropological relationship allowed me to understand both sides, which in turn helped me to keep a certain distance − a salutary posture in anthropological research − from the two groups of subjects studied, thus facilitating a critical analysis of their discourses.

Difficulties with Heuristic Benefit

In order to realise this study I needed to employ a totally neutral axiology. This was all the more necessary for the analysis as the object of my research could bring up personal convictions that had to be set aside, and as it was imperative that the subjects themselves did not feel judged. However, there are some difficulties connected to the encounter between any given problem and the methodology used to study it. Indeed, even simply telling doctors one is studying patient information risks putting them in a position where they feel the need to justify themselves, or, contrarily try to portray themselves as professionals who keep their patients 'well-informed'. All in all, there was a risk of changing their behaviour. To overcome this difficulty, it appeared productive to concentrate the first interviews with the doctors on patient behaviour, just as I choose in parallel to concentrate the first interviews with patients on doctor behaviour. Focusing the investigation on the Other helped make them less guarded about what they said.

My presence during consultations was subject to one condition: I had to wear a white coat. While I understood perfectly why the doctors imposed this condition, since patients would likely be reticent to the presence of someone other than hospital staff at the consultation, this obligation put me in a dishonest relationship which I refused to prolong thereafter. Although I was very clear about my position as a researcher at INSERM (National Institute of Health and Medical Research), it was nevertheless assumed I was part of the medical staff simply because of the coat. This caused some problematic confusion, accentuated by the fact that some doctors said that I was 'assisting' them. In truth, the patients appeared indifferent to the presence of an observer, possibly because they had other worries, and because other people are often present in the consulting room (nurses, interns, and so on). In these conditions an anthropologist, through voluntary discretion, can almost become part of the furniture. Moreover, the doctors did not always have time to make the preliminary introductions because of the frenetic pace of consultations, and the patients were not always aware of my topic of research. It is true that this knowledge could have modified how the patients behaved, since being aware of my presence and my subject would doubtless have made them monitor their attitudes more carefully. However, I chose to compensate for this lack of transparency by explaining my exact position to the patients I met again for the interview.

One of the inherent difficulties in anthropological method involving immersion, or even sometimes participation, in the situation under study, is that one's very presence can modify the conditions of observation and have a certain unintended impact. However, this simply forms part of the conditions of research and must be integrated into the analysis. In fact, the methodological and heuristic difficulties associated with the presence of an anthropologist can also have the indirect consequence of producing further information. For example, the very fact that the doctors knew about the object of the study was likely to induce them to behave differently while being observed. I noticed this effect when a patient told me: 'He didn't tell me that at the last consultation.

But when you are there, he explains things to me'. I could only manage to resolve this difficulty through a long period of study, since over time the people studied began to watch their behaviour less carefully.

Additionally, my presence at the consultations meant I had to control my own attitudes carefully because patients tend to pay attention to what is happening around them, searching for anything likely to provide them with additional information. Thus for example, during a consultation in which a patient was told that his chemotherapy had worked well and that from then on he only needed to come back for follow-up appointments, I was looking at the scans on a display board. I could see that the patient was watching me, worrying about what I could see on his scans, wondering if there was anything in particular to see there. After that experience, I made sure to look elsewhere.[11] I will return later to the topic of patients searching the words and actions of medical staff as a source of additional information. Here though, the issue is the role of the anthropologist and his/her responsibility as regards the patient's hopes of recovery. While the greatest impact in a research subject like this is obviously made with spoken words, even factors such as the observer's body language must be considered as a potential source of information. Sometimes I even had to prevent myself from giving patients a friendly smile during a consultation, since, unlike a smile exchanged during an interview, they could perceive it to be of a compassionate nature and so interpret it as a sign of the seriousness of their case.

So as not to affect the consultation process, I decided to attempt to melt into the background of the observed space and let them forget me. My position (in the space of the consulting room) was chosen so that my presence was as discrete as possible,[12] while always being visible. This concern also led me to decide not to ask questions. An anthropologist's presence is a non-presence. I realised this when I heard a couple at a consultation discussing very personal issues after the doctor left the room for a short time, and they were alone with me in the room.

The patients were informed during follow-up interviews of the fact that I was not part of the medical team. This seemed essential to me, both for ethical and methodological reasons. They were also assured of complete confidentiality, including of course the anonymity of their words. While I often had to contradict what the doctors had told them – that I was there to assist them (a precaution they deemed preferable for the patient to accept my presence), I noticed that my neutral position, or at least, my distance from the medical team, did not

---

11 But he asked me the question later when we were alone and confessed that he was wondering if they had told him the truth.

12 This did not completely remove the difficulties of my statutory position (my place in the hospital), I will return to this subject later.

displease them. On both ethical and heuristic grounds, it was important to rid myself of the medical hat they were inclined to make me wear. In practice, this meant I found myself dithering over whether to wear the white coat or not. I tried hard to make a general and neutral presentation of the object of my study – patient information – so as not to engender false responses. The spirit of the interviews was far from that of a closed questionnaire; they were designed never to induce answers such as: 'yes, I am well informed', or even 'yes, I always ask my doctor questions'. This would reveal very little considering that the problem of information is socially invested and valued in contemporary society, and that the subjects studied sometimes want to portray an image of themselves that relates to what they believe is expected of them. Therefore, I did not ask patients if they had asked any questions, or what questions they asked during a consultation, but how they felt the consultation went and what was said. Yet, given the social value assigned to asking for information in our society, even this type of neutral and very open question carries inherent bias. Indeed, I noticed such a bias when a patient told me he had asked the doctor certain questions (concerning the place where the illness 'struck', the length of the treatment and the chances of recovery) that I knew he had not, having been present at the consultation – which he probably did not remember. This reinforced my desire to observe as many interactions between patients and doctors as possible.

Establishing a relationship with informants (patients or doctors) can be complex for anthropologists since they occupy a unique position which does not necessarily fit into categories the informants recognise or into those they want to place them. The difficulty was also linked to the fact that I became a stakeholder by my very presence. I found that, despite myself, I became an actor with regards to the patients and the healthcare team. I was constantly forced to redefine my role and, above all, not let anyone think I was working *for* or *with* the doctors, a mistake that my position in the hospital could easily have engendered.

Some individuals (patients and doctors alike[13]) were confused as to the profession of anthropology, this is linked to the fact that some associate the job with that of a psychologist.[14] This produced various effects requiring mention

---

13 In this regard, I sometimes attended meetings organised by the healthcare personnel to evaluate the consultations where diagnoses are announced, where the majority of those present were psychologists who discussed their views concerning the patients' psychological reactions. My role was not to give another opinion on the subject, but to analyse what the participants were saying to understand what was at stake, as regards this issue, between the different professionals involved.

14 This confusion was clearly evident in a patient's wife's reaction in the following case: A man (a retired social security inspector) whom I asked if he would be willing to be interviewed, looked at his wife questioningly. His wife said: 'Yes, it would do you some good to talk'. (In fact, she talked just as much as he did).

here. The confusion meant that some patients assigned me a role which was not my own, but what happened as a result produced some interesting material to analyse. Although patients sometimes confused anthropology with psychology at the beginning of an interview, the confusion was quickly dissipated, but my need to rectify this for my informants[15] produced in turn other effects, notably on the role I was supposed to play in the eyes of the people under study.

Some of the patients, particularly those who saw me as the equivalent to a psychologist, reacted at first with a certain distrust that was quickly dispelled when I explained myself clearly. It seems that some people refuse to have a psychologist present because it would imply that the patient 'has a problem' – in this case, difficulty in accepting their condition. For some patients, being visited by a psychologist is tantamount to accepting that the problem lies with them, when they often want to make clear that it stems from the attitude of the doctors or the medical institution. In such circumstances, patients' refusal to see a psychologist reveals their desire for acknowledgement of the non-psychological nature of the problem. In contrast, the presence of an anthropologist allows for a different discourse, not centred on the difficulties of the patient, but on the (social or institutional) problem of information.

The discourse, thus liberated from any clinical connotations that could be interpreted as a sign that a psychological problem exists, becomes trusting and gives rise to confidences. Indeed, sometimes the patients would begin to talk saying: 'there is no point in writing that down' [this situation in fact forced me to stop taking notes, this being inappropriate behaviour when hearing secrets]. Ultimately, the patients discovered that one does not discuss the same things in the same manner with an anthropologist as with a psychologist. The interviews thus became a space for a different type of discourse. It must be noted that my role was not always clear in the eyes of the healthcare personnel either, demonstrated by psychologists or doctors asking me to collaborate with them, and wanting me to discuss what I thought of certain cases, that is to say, of certain patients, something I systematically refused to do.

My desire to make the patients understand that I was not part of the medical team was all the more important as I wanted to hear details that the patients may have chosen not to say to medical staff. But this sometimes proved difficult. This was accentuated when I was forced to ask some patients to fill out

---

15 My feeling that my presence was inappropriate sometimes made the research difficult, because unlike a psychologist, I was not there to help them, I was no use to them (even though one patient told me that she had been waiting for someone like me to tell everything to 'get it off my chest'). My uneasiness fortunately faded when the patients said they felt they had benefitted from my presence. For example, when a nurse arrived to put in a drip for a patient, I headed towards to door. The patient saw me leaving and asked me to come back to carry on talking during the process, which would take an hour, 'so that', she said, 'I can think about something else'.

a questionnaire that one of the doctors had insisted I use for my inquiries. This doctor gave his permission to carry out the study on the condition that I first handed out a questionnaire because he believed this was a method the patients were more familiar with. This involved asking them forcedly rigid questions, sometimes with very little bearing on the particular context within which their history was placed. Apart from the limits inherent in using questionnaires that do not fulfil the requirements of qualitative research, it was problematic in this case because distributing them while wearing a white coat reinforced the confusion over my role, leading patients to assume that I was part of the medical body. This was evident in one man's comment added to the bottom of the questionnaire: 'I would like to take advantage of this questionnaire to compliment the healthcare team at all levels', convinced as he was that the questionnaire was issued by the hospital services.

The uncertain situation I found myself in − I was sometimes considered to be an outsider to the hospital, sometimes a member of the healthcare team, on the part of both patients and healthcare workers − is evident in the following examples. During one consultation I attended, the doctor and then the nurse left the room. The nurse came back to write out the prescription of a treatment and said to me: 'Oh, you are taking notes! Did he specify the dosage?' (I assessed the unwarranted position she put me in, and did not feel entitled to tell her what the doctor had said). Another example: after the doctor had explained the treatment he had prescribed to the patient, he left, as did the nurse assisting him. The patient then asked if I was going to prescribe the treatment. I replied that I wasn't. This type of situation is detrimental in several ways: not only in ethical terms, as the white coat that the doctor obliged me to wear in order to be present at the consultation had led the patient to believe that I was part of the medical team and had made me complicit in the deception organised by the doctor,[16] but also in epistemological terms: this biased the information that patients could provide me with, since, perceived to be part of the medical body, I could not then be trusted with information not given to the doctors. It was thus also for methodological reasons that I needed to correct this false image assigned to me.

Once the informants had understood that anthropologists are not psychologists, nor doctors, nor nurses, the next inevitable question was: What then are they for? Although I clearly explained that my work was not associated in any way with the healthcare personnel, several patients asked me questions which revealed the diversity of expectations they had of me. Another patient once asked me: 'Since you are in the profession, can you recommend someone who practices holistic medicine and is interested in the body as a whole?

---

16   That is why I made my exact position clear at every opportunity − particularly when I met patients outside the consulting room.

An anthroposophist or something like that? That is what you do, isn't it? Because in France, the doctors are only interested in organs, but they don't look any further!' I replied that that was not what I did and that I had little knowledge in the area. So he said: 'Can I be critical? You are just like the doctors, you do not try to understand alternative types of medicine!!' One patient, an environmental activist, to whom I explained my reasons for being in the service, replied: 'Ah! I've been waiting for someone like you! There are so many things I want to ask you: Who is doing research on dioxins in the blood? Why do the researchers not make their results available? Why do they not look at levels of radioactivity in people? And why are we not informed about dioxins that are teratogenic and cancerogenic? And what about farmer's wives and pesticides? They are always hiding everything. They hid Chernobyl from us, they lie all the time'. Another difficulty of my particular position became apparent when patients tried to obtain information on their case through me, obliging me to become an actor in the process of acquiring information concerning them.

Finally, it is necessary to mention a difficulty which proved, against all odds, to bring a real heuristic benefit. I was sometimes missing certain information about the patients I had seen during consultations. Notably, for several of them, I did not know their socioprofessional backgrounds. In some cases, I was able to ask them later when I saw them again, but for those I did not meet again, I lacked this information. Some doctors subsequently gave it to me, others refused to do so, and would not give me permission to look in their files.

However, I quickly realised that very often the doctors did not know either. 'I have too many patients, I don't have the time to look at that', they sometimes told me, even while agreeing to give me the information. The frenetic pace of the consultations, often up to 25 in a morning, did not allow them the time to search for this information in the files, when it was there at all. And so, I could only guess at the social position of these patients and gather a rough idea of their social background from external signs, such as language, clothing, bodily attitudes and so on, all approximate signs indicating their social belonging. Nevertheless, this left me uncertain as to their socioprofessional affiliation, since sociocultural level is often unrelated to socioeconomic position.

I realised however that the doctors who had not taken the time to look for this information in the patients' files found themselves in a situation similar to mine, and I noticed that despite themselves, they were also searching for social indicators in their patients. As we will see, it turned out that their behaviour changes with different patients not just in function to their social background, that is to say not just according to who the patients *are*, but in function to who the doctor *thinks they are*, a judgement made through reading external signs. Although at the beginning, being denied information relating to the socioprofessional background of certain patients appeared to be a significant methodological handicap, it actually became an asset to the extent that it allowed me pinpoint a reality which was to become one of the fundamental aspects of the results of this research.

In the first two parts of this book, I will examine the reality of information for the actors and those around them (the healthcare team for the doctors, and close friends and family for the patients), before addressing the question of lying on both sides. This division acknowledges the fact that some realities relating to the problem of information do not pertain to lying and must be treated separately. Moreover, the work aims to shed light on lying by 'zooming in', to the extent that lying can only be distinguished, in many respects, from non-information by the degree to which it is practiced. In terms of doctor's lies, I will examine how the doctors justify the lies they tell, the ethical and therapeutic options underlying their choices, the doctrine built by health professionals on this subject, and also the similarities and differences between lying and keeping secrets.

For good measure, I will examine not only the way in which patients perceive the information they receive (on the diagnosis, the prognosis or the treatment), but also what information they themselves give the doctors, notably concerning their treatments, their therapeutic choices, the symptoms they detect and the pain they experience. We will see that, on both sides, the discourses are not homogenous and that various logics underpin the behaviours of the subjects. This heterogeneity however does not exclude recurrent mechanisms. We will see how these work and what they mean.

In the third part, I will further examine some dimensions that characterise exchanges between doctors and patients. These dimensions reveal the existence of numerous 'misunderstandings', the origins of which I will attempt to unearth. From this, I will also critically appraise the issue of communication between doctors and patients, the decision-making power of the latter, and the nature of the medical relationship within which lying appears to be an intractable ingredient.

Chapter 1
The Doctors

Doctors and Information

I will attempt here, by examining the explanations and comments of doctors on one hand, to decipher the ethical positions they purport to hold and the justifications they give for their behaviour, and through observation of their attitudes during consultations on the other hand, to discover what mechanisms their practices of providing or not providing information to patients are objectively based on. The issue of information will be considered from two different angles: firstly through a discussion of general information on the affliction in question and its treatments, and then by using information concerning the patient's particular case, because, as we will see, the issue of information in doctor–patient relationships continually oscillates between these two registers. There exists a wide variety of attitudes concerning information provision: from doctors who tell their patients almost nothing, just the bare legal minimum, to those who tell them everything, in order to protect themselves from the possibility of prosecution. The majority however only provide some of the information they possess. The aim is thus to find out what they say, what type of things they reveal and do not reveal, to whom and under what conditions.

It is generally accepted amongst health professionals today that 'the diagnosis is almost never withheld from the patient'. On learning the subject of this research, an intern stated with conviction: 'Whether to say it or not applies to the prognosis. Because the diagnosis is no longer a problem; we talk freely about cancer nowadays!' This conviction, shared almost unanimously by doctors today, should be considered as a preconception since, with closer observation, it is evident that while many doctors claim to be in favour of patient information and are convinced that this information is now fully provided, the reality in practice is that this information is not so freely given.

The majority of doctors agree that not everything should be revealed to a patient. They set certain limits to this information and apply conditions to its provision. In this way, the doctors have created a doctrine to which they adhere almost unanimously − although some variations can nevertheless be observed. For example, doctors assume it is obvious that patients should only be informed if they want to be. 'We only truly inform patients in response to a request', said one oncologist. Another said: 'I only say such things in answer to a clear and precise question'. 'The degree of precision I give depends on the degree of precision of the questioning', clarified another. However, although all doctors chant this doctrinal principle in unison, this attitude is obviously problematic to the extent that, as this research reveals, many patients say they do not know what or how to ask. Thus the question is, how do the doctors detect the existence of a request for such information on the part of the patients?

The doctors cite two main types of obstacle to information provision. The first is linked to the difficulty of making patients understand that, while they can be informed of their diagnosis, this cannot be done for their prognosis.

Indeed, it is commonly thought that information cannot be provided on the prognosis since the doctors cannot actually predict the patient's future, how their disease will progress and what will become of their health status. 'Some people not only want to know their diagnosis but also their prognosis. That is much harder, because we can't tell them that, we really don't know', one doctor remarked. This observation refers to the degree of uncertainty that exists on the subject of prognosis, a difficulty well known to health professionals. Aside from the psychological and existential difficulties inherent in telling patients that their health is deteriorating or that they might die, it is often this uncertainty that is at the heart of the doctor's reluctance to provide a prognosis.

While some doctors cite the law as a reason for saying everything, fearing the excesses of an increasingly litigious society, others choose to limit the information they provide to that which is certain. In making a prognosis, doctors risk making a mistake and maximising the risks incurred by giving false information or by making a statement that the patient takes to be information, when the doctor does not. This uncertainty thus takes us to the problem of knowing what can be said and under what conditions, which is even more challenging for the prognosis than the diagnosis. But, as we will see, the problem becomes even more complicated when there is no clear boundary between the diagnosis and the prognosis.

The issue of information hinges on that of truth even though it can evidently not be reduced simply to that. However, many professionals do not believe that the problem can be perceived in terms of truth and lies, precisely because of the uncertainty surrounding how the disease will develop. 'Anyway, it is never possible to tell the truth. Even if we are sure that the patient is done for, we wouldn't say: "you only have 3 months left"! We could always get it wrong, we are not God', explained one doctor. 'Truth doesn't exist', said another, 'we can never be sure of recognising the truth'. However, this type of argument is specious in that many of the practices of information retention, or even lying, cannot be explained by this uncertainty. Indeed, there are some things that hold true at a certain point in time given the knowledge available, which may subsequently be supplanted by another truth as medical advances are made. And the truth concerning a patient's health status and the present evolution of his/her affliction does in fact exist. The uncertainty simply underlines the temporary character of the truth, it does not eliminate the real contents of this knowledge. Thus, a distinction must be made between the truth as an unknowable reality and the truth as the reality one believes to be true. Therefore, the argument of uncertainty only applies to the prognosis and not to the diagnosis nor to the known effects of a treatment for example. As such it is appropriate to raise the question of truth, not simply in terms of reality, but also in terms of what we think reality is or what we actually know of it, and to distinguish between the posture that refuses to predict what is not known and the posture that refuses to say what is known. Only the second posture is relevant to the issue of patient information. Using the argument of uncertainty obscures the existence of situations in which doctors possess knowledge but nevertheless do not communicate it to patients, but this does not exhaust the problem of trying to identify the mechanisms inherent in not providing information and in telling lies.

The diagnosis and the prognosis are two distinct stages in the overall process of making statements concerning the afflictions of patients. While the diagnosis is relatively easy in that it can be made by reading the results of various examinations (ultrasound, scan, blood tests for example), the prognosis, on the other hand, is the result of a *judgement* (itself made using objective data) on the probable outcome of the illness. It thus relies on suppositions and deductions and is based on logical reasoning and the statistical data available on the development of the disease.

The second difficulty the doctors mentioned, which is partly linked to the problem of uncertainty, concerns the statistical truth of information. The difficulty lies in getting the patient to accept that the only information that can be provided on a prognostic level is statistical, which in fact has no direct bearing on a particular individual case. 'I can't say whether this is a cancer you recover from, because even if you have a type of cancer with a 90 per cent survival rate, I can't know if you are in the 10 per cent or the 90 per cent' one doctor attempted to explain to his patient to make her understand his reluctance to provide statistical information. Here again, the doctors very often avoid the problem of truth, believing that their patients have not understood the exclusively statistical value of their prospects for recovery when they accuse the doctors of not telling the truth. 'People say we are lying to them when we tell them they have a good chance of recovery, because they are not in fact getting better!' But we will see that lying results from very different mechanisms, and that the problem here is that of the difference in scales between doctors' and patients' discourses.

Ethical and therapeutic options

The issues of information and truth are difficult to dissociate. Here some preliminary considerations are presented in order to introduce the arguments doctors make to justify the way they conceive and manage the provision of information to patients. This discussion will be taken further when examining the links between doctors and lying.

The ethical dimension of the issue of information and truth has been widely debated in the literature (Cassileth 1979; Bok 1979; Fletcher 1979). These authors all highlighted the ethical dilemma of whether to tell the truth or lie. In reference to the Hippocratic Oath which says that one must do the patient no harm, some take this dictate as a reason not to reveal to patients their health status or their prognosis. Others use this same dictate to mean that one should not withhold information from the people it concerns. 'Do no harm' is a relatively subjective judgement.

Cassileth (1979) showed that informed patients deal with and understand therapeutic measures better. Others recommend that doctors keep genuine information to themselves in the name of 'therapeutic privilege' on the grounds that 'with uncertainty, comes hope' (MacIntosh 1979).[1] These doctors believe that revealing an illness is equivalent to giving a death sentence (Oken 1961), while some authors see their silence to be the result of the doctors' own fear of death (Konior and Levine 1975).

Given that the debate is framed in ethical terms, the supporters of truth often construct their opinions in response to positions advocated by its detractors and formulate their justifications on the same ground as the latter. Thus, in response to the argument sometimes made by the doctors to justify not providing information, which says it is better to remain silent to lessen the patient's suffering, Katz (1984) argued that to the contrary, silence produces negative effects and causes suffering in patients, and that information is a therapeutic necessity because it relieves suffering. He made a strong plea in support of the truth and its power to liberate patients from isolation. Similarly, in a challenge to his colleagues who believe one should withhold the truth in order to protect patients from the fear of death and ensure the best possible attitude to fight the disease, Abiven (1996) declared that 'the truth is less difficult to accept than the anxiety induced by secrets' and argued that the practice of lying 'to do good' or 'to be humane' is the true cause of suffering.

The issue of truth remains a major aspect of the ethical debates on the treatment of patients, especially cancer patients. The ethical positions are themselves supported by philosophical positions: while Kant believed that truth is an absolute and unconditional must, Benjamin Constant however proposed the existence of the 'right to lie, for benevolent motives'.[2]

---

1   The terms 'therapeutic privilege' or 'therapeutic exception' allow doctors to hide information that could harm the patient (Bolly et al).

2   Although it was developed in the political context of the French Revolution, Benjamin Constant's position can be, and is, applied to other contexts. For example, Cyril Morana discussed

Following in the same philosophical vein as Kant, Fletcher (1979) thinks the idea that it is sometimes good to lie is unjustifiable and that the truth is essential to our democratic ideal. He highlighted the dangers of not revealing the truth by evoking the case of a patient who asked his doctor never to tell him if ever he was seriously ill. Fletcher asked: 'Later on, what will he think when his doctor gives him reassuring news? He may truly believe that his illness is not serious and that he is being told the truth, but the doctor may be following his initial request, in which case, he is lying'. Fletcher concluded that this would cause a disastrous situation. His example is thus an illustration not only of a moral situation but also of a logical one, since the patient finds himself in the same state of perplexity as the person hearing Epimenides' message in his famous paradox.

Supporters and detractors of the truth have thus developed numerous arguments (see Geets 1993),[3] but what is most striking is that the same arguments ('for the good of the patient' or 'to do the patient no harm') are used to support radically opposing positions.

However, the authors of publications on this subject are not the only ones to discuss this question. Faced with the imperative to inform patients, doctors themselves also confront such ethical questions. For example, they ask themselves: 'How can I tell patients their condition is deteriorating without making them panic or become demoralised?' or, when the prognosis leaves no hope: 'How can I make patients understand that they will be moving from curative treatment to palliative care?' The dilemma faced by doctors is linked to the conflict inherent in trying to follow two distinct and sometimes antagonistic principles: the principle of non-maleficence (a variation of the principle of beneficence), which is the basis of the decision to say nothing so as not to let the patient lose hope, and the principle of autonomy (Reich 2004).[4]

At this first stage, we could qualify the state of tension experienced by the doctors stemming from a simultaneous reference to two partly contradictory ethical principles as 'ethical dissonance'. They must, on one hand, reassure

---

a lie told to the Nazis to save someone's life, and says that lying is authorised in this case because the person being lied to is not 'deserving of the truth'. Therefore, as Constant (2003) said: 'One is only obliged to tell the truth to those who have the right to it; but no man has the right to truth when he harms others'.

3 Some believe that patients will be empowered by knowing their affliction and will discover there a reason to actively cooperate with their doctor, others think that an atmosphere of deception can lead patients to exaggerate the gravity of their affliction, which exacerbates their anxiety (Geets 1993).

4 The question is also raised when it is not the doctor but the patient's family who do not want the patient to be told his/her diagnosis, or the prognosis if it is bad. On this subject Mr Reich asked: 'Is it ethically justifiable and acceptable to accept the family's stance and not divulge the diagnosis or prognosis?'

the patient (a role some attribute to the paternalistic model of doctor–patient relations), and on the other, allow them autonomy, or in other words, give patients their liberty and let them manage their own lives and bodies (this role fits into a more egalitarian relationship). Yet, the issue of patient information mobilises these two partly contradictory principles, placing the doctor in a sort of double bind. The model of egalitarian relationships nonetheless appears inadequate to those who cannot see how patients can possibly take decisions concerning their health. The model of shared decision-making advocated by some health professionals in order to defend patient information, is disputed by others, who perceive this to be more the beginning of a model of 'shared anxiety'. After having revealed the inherent risks of a proposed treatment to a patient, a doctor said bitterly:

> I have to tell him, it is the law; besides, in my letter to colleagues which includes a consultation report, I am obliged to write 'in agreement with the patient' or 'duly informed' … There is a social pressure to say everything even if the risk is 1 in 100,000. Why worry patients when they could die anyway of renal or heart failure if I don't give them this treatment? I am not in control anymore. Today, we no longer practice a paternalistic style but a contractual style of medicine; if they want shared decision-making, they get shared anxiety as well! We no longer have the right to prescribe carcinogenic drugs without saying so, when the risk is only theoretical! In fact, for them, letting them decide means they can decide between the drawbacks of cortisone and the drawbacks of the disease itself.

Some doctors however come to question whether the reassuring role they try to adopt when refusing to give a patient bad news is actually a good thing, or at the very least, they put the advantages in perspective: 'One day, I had to tell a woman the results of her biopsy by telephone. She phoned and I confirmed her diagnosis (she had liver metastases) in a very comforting way; too comforting! Because after that, it was very difficult to make her come in quickly for the treatment, which need to be started urgently. She said, "if it's not serious, there's no need to rush"'.

Medical arguments

Various and contrasting mechanisms exist that dictate the choices made among the health professionals who advocate patient information. Their reasons for making this argument are not always the same, and mean they take differing ethical positions. On this subject, the doctor population is divided between those who advocate information *in itself* (the patient's right to know) and information *for a determined end*; that is information as a means of convincing patients of the necessity of following a certain treatment.[5] In the first case, it is a matter of informing patients as people with the right to know about matters concerning them and their bodies; in the second case, information is considered necessary so that patients adhere better to their treatment regime or sometimes *only if* this would encourage patients to accept the treatment.[6] The first position advocates a principle, the second takes a practical stance. The principled position and the practical one borrow from distinct registers: the first takes a moral approach, the second a medical one. The therapeutic necessity of information is very clearly expressed by this doctor: 'When chemotherapy is required, I provide all the information because it is necessary since there will be a treatment evaluation; therefore, the patient must be informed of it'. In these circumstances, he provides information for practical, functional and utilitarian reasons. 'I tell them if the treatment doesn't work just so they understand the need to change the protocol'. Practical information provision is more a therapeutic strategy than an ethical or philosophical option.[7]

The problem becomes particularly thorny when a conflict arises between ethical and therapeutic options. Yet, by examining the reasons behind doctors' decisions to say or not say, we can see that they sometimes collide, and that the doctors find themselves faced with a Cornelian dilemma between therapeutic options and ethical ones. Indeed, it is clear that there can be a risk of not even reaching a diagnosis, even in serious cases, because the patient is not sufficiently worried and will not agree to therapy. In these circumstances doctors can find themselves torn since for ethical reasons they may believe that the truth should not be told but for therapeutic reasons they may think it should be. Whether to admit to the seriousness of the situation and spell out the patient's possible future can become a therapeutic decision and be part of a methodology: information provision is seen as a tool in aid of therapy; it aims to create a situation in which patients take responsibility for their own health and accept the medical recommendations they are given. Conversely, when doctors perceive a patient's future to be completely hopeless and there are no more therapeutic decisions to be made, they may still refuse to inform a patient of his/her diagnosis out of

---

5   In the course of their professional experience, all the doctors I spoke to have had cases where they have had to assess the risks involved in under-informing patients on their health status. An appreciation of the potential harm inherent in under-informing is precisely what leads some of them to advocate the need to inform for practical ends.

6   We should maybe question whether the therapeutic justification alone for providing information is relevant for the doctors if we take into account the conclusions of several studies that show very little correlation between the degree of knowledge of a disease and the degree to which treatments are adhered to (Meichenbaum and Turk 1987).

7   In *Mourir*, a novel by Schnitzler, the seriously ill protagonist is told by his spouse that the doctor is lying 'just to scare you, so you will be more careful'. Here, it is the lie that is utilitarian.

a conviction of the social futility of the statement.[8] Others, on the other hand, think that the very absence of therapeutic considerations, when the patient's behaviour will have no effect on their health status, means the patient should be informed so they can 'organise themselves' and 'put their affairs in order' before they die. In this case it is the social or therapeutic use of information that dictates behaviour concerning the disclosure of a diagnosis or prognosis.

The information that doctors give patients is extremely variable and concerns as much the diagnosis as the prognosis or the proposed treatments and their expected effects, adverse side-effects or risks. However, doctors most often identify the issue of information with that of disclosing the diagnosis. The direct link between these two issues is that revealing the truth is often judged to be too harsh, and that it is necessary to codify the way in which the disclosure is made in order to lessen the shock. Delaporte (2001) thus called for moderation, and denounced the fact that doctors end up being harsh in the name of truth, although she also condemned 'filtered' truth which opens the door to anxiety.

There is a thriving debate in France today on the issue of disclosure and the procedure that has been put in place (though still in an experimental stage) for revealing serious diagnoses following the demands of patient associations. This question is being addressed by numerous committees and is the object of a great many recommendations and meetings, some of which I was able to attend and on which I will make some comments here. The majority of specialists agree that 'the announcement does not need to be long but it must be discussed several times. Repetition is more important than length'. Some prefer to talk of an 'announcement procedure' rather than an 'announcement', such as Henri Pujol, President of the *Ligue nationale contre le cancer*, who said: 'The information process is a continuous process; we cannot say: "I informed a patient between 12:00 and 12:40". The patient may want to know one thing one day and something else the next. It is this process we are referring to in the phrase "announcement procedure"'. The provision of information by doctors is in fact the object of various guidelines within hospital departments according

---

8 It is easy to conceive of a doctor's reluctance to tell a patient about a risk he believes he has to take in order to avoid taking another, bigger, one. The doctor has to make a *risk calculation* he may not think appropriate to share with the patient. For example, a doctor explained to a patient suffering from a stenosis increased with a massive phlebothrombosis: 'Your oesophagus is constricted, there may be lesions which cause bleeding. I would like to see if there are any, without a general anaesthetic. A small clot could go into the lung and create a pulmonary embolism, so I need to give you anti-coagulants. I will give you heparin'. But in the hallway he added to his students: 'There is phlebitis which goes up into the pelvis. If it is a malignant oesophagitis, giving him Heparin will put him in great risk; there is a risk of a serious embolism, a risk of death, even within 10 minutes. But there is also the risk of cardiac arrest, therefore a general anaesthetic would also be very risky, so it is not possible to do a colonoscopy; otherwise that would have been ideal'.

to which, for example, information should be given in stages in response to patient's questions.

As this procedure implies, and as the *Plan Cancer* recognises in its recommendations, the notion of 'announcement' in the singular holds little relevance since if patients and their afflictions are considered over time, it is evident that their stories are marked by a series of announcements – the announcement of the presence of the disease when it is discovered and identified, but also, announcements concerning its development or developments, both in quantitative terms (for example the growth of a tumour) and in qualitative terms (its displacement towards another organ) – and that the truth can only be revealed progressively. Indeed, the health professionals themselves stress the need to take patients towards the truth very gently. We will see later that, alongside this process of truth in stages, there also exists what we could call lying in stages.

Among the guidelines given to doctors that most oncologists integrate into their doctrine, is the necessity of not leaving the patient with a negative fact: 'if we announce bad news, we must follow that straight away with a discussion of the treatment', the oncologists explain. In fact, they generally discuss the possible treatments just after having announced the bad diagnosis, following the guideline which says one should not leave a patient with sad news. An oncologist said to his patient: 'Unfortunately the cells have become resistant. We need to find another treatment'. (Then straight after he said): 'There are two other possibilities that could be effective. Nothing is certain. There is one based on classic chemotherapy, and a newer treatment, using a new antibody, which goes to the cancer targets and blocks the evolution. But, for it to be effective, we have to be sure that your cells really do express the target of this antibody. We need to do some tests. Eighty per cent of the cases are positive. If you are in the 20 per cent who do not express the target of this antibody, we will use chemotherapy'. We will see however that the implementation of the 'announcement consultation' and the recommendations it carries are contested by some doctors who believe that each individual case is unique so the announcement cannot be standardised (see Lévy-Soussan 2004).

The 'announcement consultation' aside, not all doctors unanimously agree on the need to make an announcement at all. Some think it is completely pointless to be explicit on this subject, since 'they know anyway'. They believe that the question of knowing what should be said to patients is a false debate since 'the patient already knows'. 'In fact, there is never really an announcement, since patients already suspect the truth when they come to the consultations. They have already done the tests, x-rays, and so on. At some point they are sure'. Such knowledge, which is sometimes borne out by the fact the patients already know their test results before the consultation with the oncologist, is perceived as a vague knowledge, based on a supposition which contains no objectifiable element, which doctors express as a feeling. They believe the patient 'feels' it, and they attribute to their patients a sort of prescience on their health status to justify their belief that there is no point to giving them clear and explicit information. They justify their silence about the diagnosis when it is bad in this way. 'There is no need to tell patients that they have lots of metastases! They know it anyway', said one doctor. Therefore, using the argument that patients already know what is wrong with them, the doctors not only think it is totally useless to inform them but also absolve themselves of failing to inform by referring to this vague knowledge that patients have of their affliction. Finally, the idea that this knowledge is not worth sharing is occasionally based on the idea that patients sometimes know a lot more than the doctors themselves: 'the announcement, the announcement! Sometimes it is the patient who announces a recurrence to me!'

Although they are convinced that patients are told everything, many doctors use all sorts of strategies to avoid saying things clearly. By observing the consultations, I identified various techniques to lessen the shock of discovering a diagnosis or a test result. The most frequent strategy employed is the tendency to play down the affliction in order to make the situation less daunting. One oncologist recommends: 'it is better to say: "you have a large polyp which could become cancerous" than "you have cancer"; it is better for patients to suggest the danger than to terrorise them'. Indeed, I observed this technique of minimisation during the consultations. It can also be done by using terms intending to reduce the problem: 'we need to do more chemo because there is a *little* nodule in the lungs, and we need to do something to stop it growing', one doctor said to his patient. This mechanism involves imparting the diagnosis of the disease or its development using euphemisms: 'There are these *tiny little* things: nodules in the lung and liver; we need to use another treatment and target these cells with chemotherapy'. However, once this consultation was over and the patient had left, the oncologist dictated the consultation report specifying the existence of a 'large mass on the lung'. Sometimes the diagnosis is told clearly, without beating around the bush. But then, it may be the treatment that is described in euphemisms. After receiving the results of a biopsy, an oncologist told his patient: 'it is cancer, we are going to start a *little bit* of chemo'. In his view, the announcement of a treatment induces more fear than the one for the diagnosis.

However, half-said announcements fool no one. The terms used to talk about cancer or a tumour without saying the actual words have the same emotional impact on the patient: 'the urologist didn't tell me much. He didn't directly say I had cancer, but he led me to understand that I did. He said: "there is something but we need to do more tests to be sure". I understood'. To say the word 'something', is the same as saying 'cancer' or 'tumour'. It is the word that says without saying, and becomes a category that all fears can be attached to.

'Instead of using the word cancer, I say "multiplication" or "run away" cells that are "out of control"', an oncologist explained. 'Instead of saying chemo, I talk of a medical treatment. Why frighten them when we can use circumlocutions?'

Although most doctors, as we have seen, develop relatively consensual strategies on how to behave with patients in order to conform to the law but without nevertheless saying too much, some however develop very personal strategies: 'I am always positive. If the patients ask me if it is serious, I say yes. If they ask me if they will recover, I say yes as well. That means that is what they want to hear'. Others do not have a fixed strategy, but let themselves be guided by the specific situation: 'I work by intuition; I go on my instincts'. Others again do not see the use of worrying about the way the diagnosis is disclosed. 'Anyhow, there is no good way of announcing bad news!' one oncologist said.

Within this group, some take no precautions at all. In fact, not all doctors care about sparing their patients' feelings, and the message can sometimes be very harsh. One patient, who had delayed going to her doctor after having found a lump in her breast, said: 'When the doctor saw me in the consultation, his reaction was: "Honestly! Have you seen how gross your breast looks?! Why didn't you come earlier? I am going to try and save it but nothing is certain!"'. Psychologists interpret such harshness by doctors as a reflection of the doctor's own uneasiness: 'If a doctor announces news in a harsh way, it is because he himself has a problem with death', explained the psychologist of an oncology department. But in this we can also see a reflection of the fact that some doctors are not happy that they have less freedom than before to decide on the information they provide to patients and whether to tell the truth or not, because of a law partly drafted through patient demands. In this category we can place doctors whose behaviour with patients seems to be the result of a bitterness towards what the law obliges them to do. After a consultation in which a doctor had bluntly told his patient that her cancer was very advanced, he said to me: 'They wanted the truth, didn't they? They even got themselves a law for it! Well, here it is!'

Sometimes, patients discover information concerning them when their doctor dictates a letter to a colleague or makes a consultation report by speaking into a Dictaphone in the patients' presence. Thus the information is transmitted indirectly, mediated by an object since the doctor is not talking directly to the patient but to a colleague or simply a medical secretary charged with transcribing the information to put in the patient's files. In such a case, doctors sometimes say things they had not necessarily told the patient previously and that the patient discovers in this way. There is obviously no general rule on this subject: some doctors systematically dictate their letters in front of patients; others always do it in their absence (for example in the corridor, having left the consulting room); others again use different strategies depending on the case. One dictates his letters and consultation reports in front of patients when he knows them and thinks he 'knows' that they can hear the contents of the letter, but dictates them in the corridor when he does not know them and so does not know how they might react on hearing their exact diagnosis stated, or when he is in doubt, so as not to cause any undue anxiety. Moreover, when patients come to a consultation through a referral by a colleague, many doctors prefer to write a letter to their colleague without informing the patient of their diagnosis, or refuse to answer the questions patients ask. (Some doctors refuse to give patients this information on the pretext that it is necessary to avoid infringing the principle of reciprocity which says that a doctor consulted on the advice of a GP should not 'steal' their patients but should send them and the information concerning them back.)[9]

It is common, despite their obligation to inform patients, for doctors to offload to the family information they should be giving the patient. 'Sometimes, the patient's family ask me questions. I am much more open with the family. I am more likely to say the patient is not doing well. I say: "It is not going too well, I am worried". It is important for the family to know and they don't generally tell the patient'. On the other hand, doctors can sometimes find themselves in a position of complicity with the family who want the information to be withheld from the patient: 'One shouldn't say very different things to the family and the patient; at the same time, I don't want to mistreat the family by not saying anything and sometimes they want to hide things from the patient'. Conversely, doctors sometimes find themselves in conflict with patients' families who do not want them to be told the truth when the doctors themselves would like them to be told.

Added to the idea that 'anyhow, they already know what is wrong with them', which is at the base of the opinion of some doctors that there is no point in informing the patient, as discussed above, comes the conviction that when patients do not know something 'all they have to do is ask'. Here it is a matter not simply of an illusion of information, but an illusion of the ease in which it can be obtained. 'If they want a certain piece of information, they can always get it; whether it concerns the diagnosis or the therapy'. However, doctors do not always like being questioned. Some see it as a sign of a lack of trust: 'Some patients trust me, others don't; they ask lots of questions; it's a question of personality!'

In reality, the idea that patients do not want to know is very widespread in the medical environment. This idea totally contradicts what the patients say – they claim that no-one wants to tell them anything. If we look at this a little deeper and try to understand the basis on which doctors deduce their patient's desire to know or not, we find the phrase: 'If people do not ask questions, it is simple, we say nothing. If they are not asking, we shouldn't say

---

9   On 'sending patients back', see Sarradon-Eck et al. (2004).

anything. If they don't ask, it is because they don't want to know'. In the name of protecting them, health professionals advocate a new right for patients: the right not to know.

Equally, many authors (Geets 1993, for example) believe that the right to the truth should go hand in hand with the right not to know.[10] Likewise, Bensaïd (1981) thinks that 'in almost every case, the truth is there, available to those who want it'. This right to not know is reaffirmed by Massé (2003) who considers that the public health system has a moral responsibility to respect citizens' rights to trust experts to make decisions for them when giving up their right to informed consent. Or, in order to justify patient misunderstanding of inadequate or fragmented information, some doctors take refuge behind psychological analyses such as 'patients understand what they want to'. In maintaining that patients do not want to know, doctors often ascribe to them an expectation they do not have,[11] just as they underestimate, according to Vennin et al. (1995), the desire women with breast cancer have for their families to be informed (Pierret 1998). The quality of the information provided is barely questioned, and rarely is it considered that patients may have a good capacity to understand on the condition that they are provided with the necessary elements, even when they do not dare ask for them. One oncologist explained: 'Some patients ask a lot. For example, they want to know what segment of the liver the nodule is in. While others ask nothing at all! They are in complete denial!' The equivalence he makes between the lack of questions and denial reveals a total negligence of the fact that some patients do not know how to ask the right questions. To say, as one oncologist did, 'if patients don't ask questions, it is because they don't want to know, they are scared of the answer', is to totally deny the sociological dimension of verbal exchanges between doctors and patients. It is interesting to stress that in the field, doctors claimed with conviction that certain patients 'don't want to know', when those same patients asked me to find information out for them because they did not know how, or did not dare, to ask for themselves. Practitioners sometimes take patients' words at face value, as the words of this oncologists show: 'The proof that they don't want to know, is that they often say, "doctor, tell me it is not serious"!' This phrase does not necessarily mean that the patient does not want to know the truth, it could just as well be interpreted to mean, 'Doctor, please do something to make it not serious', equivalent to a means of warding off the disease by hoping that the doctor will assure them of their favourable chances of recovery.

---

10   Geets (1993) said: 'If few patients express a desire to know the truth, it is either because they do not want to know, or because they already know, more or less'.

11   Following a mechanism fairly similar to that in which GPs assume patients have a strong expectation of obtaining medicines in order to justify their overabundant prescriptions.

This idea is the subject of a complete consensus in the medical setting. One doctor explained: 'Most of the time, the patients don't want to know. For example, I saw a patient yesterday with lots of metastases on the liver and lung and she knows it. But she came in saying: "You know doctor, I have an iron constitution, I will live to 100!" She obviously doesn't want to know and it's not my place to tell her'. With these words, the oncologist shows his refusal to take account of the performative nature of the patient's words. However, here again, we could just as well conclude that her words do not mean she is refusing her diagnosis, but that knowing it does not stop her from wanting to convince herself that it is not life threatening – this is not the same thing.

It is appropriate to note here the omnipresence of psychological analysis in the medical field, and that this type of analysis is much more widely spread than any other human science. The psychological approach to the problem (see for example Ruszniewski 1995) is what leads actors to systematically explain patients' lack of questions in terms of denial, or refusal to know the truth, and to ignore the fact that, very often, patients do not dare ask their oncologist questions, while they are obviously looking to gather the information from the nursing staff or in the media. But this statement (and the analysis underpinning it) also allows doctors to avoid re-evaluating their attitude to patients, since they believe that if the patient does not have access to information, it is because they do not want it.

While they recognise that some patients want to know as much as possible about their illness, the doctors become alarmed, even angry, when they hear that these patients are trying to gather information from other sources. In particular, patients can be strongly reprimanded by their doctors when their desire for information, barely sated during interactions with health professionals responsible for their care, leads them to search for information on the Internet. Doctors generally take it very badly when patients resort to the Internet. Their worries can be legitimate however since some patients are incapable of critically evaluating the source of the information they find:

> There is one category of difficult patients: teachers, doctors and researchers because they have an intellectual knowledge base which means they think they can understand things that they don't in fact grasp. They go on the Internet which is a disaster because they don't filter the information. For example, one woman had read on the Internet that running without a bra caused cancer. It may be true that it can cause micro-tears and that the breasts can fall faster, but it in no way causes cancer! They ask questions about the treatments and their side-effects and they make life difficult for themselves. Just like the leaflets listing all the side-effects! The laboratories provide them for legal reasons, but too much information drowns information! And then we can no longer see the two or three most important effects. Informing people is not necessarily being honest!

Hardey (2004) explained the dangers of the Internet when users do not differentiate the contents and rightly shows how the architecture of the Internet means one click takes you from an informative site to a commercial one. (But isn't there also a risk for doctors, who are faced with large amounts of information from medical journals and medical representatives, to not be able to discriminate between informative discourse and marketing?) One intern told a hospitalised patient and his wife: 'You mustn't believe what you read or hear about this, whether in journals, on the Internet or elsewhere. We are the only ones you should believe!' (We will see how patients take such advice later).

Convinced that only some patients want to know but aware that not all communication is verbal, some doctors attempt to decipher the patients' demand for information through other signs: 'Some we can spot from the beginning by the way they look at us'. Here, the doctors are looking for clues from their patients that reflect a desire to know the truth. For example, doctors analyse the patient's expression to find out what they should say, demonstrating their attention to infra-verbal language: 'There is information in a look, not just in words. Silences sometimes allow us to find out what the patient wants'. The doctors thus develop techniques for sounding out a desire for information. Many say it is a case of 'feeling' the patient's request for information.[12] Here we should note the arbitrary nature of feeling as a subjective evaluation of the needs of others.[13] This recommendation also turns up in sociological writing. Bataille (2003) recommends that doctors do not go 'further than people can cope with', expressing the position of the *Ligue nationale contre le cancer* and of oncologists campaigning for this strategy. Indeed, health professionals agree that when patients find the information they are given distressing, they are often too stunned to take in any additional information and then think they have not been fully informed and become increasingly anxious and depressed (Ong et al. 1995).

Here the aim is not to reject this type of analysis but to show that the issue of information cannot simply be reduced to a psychological perspective and to propose another one that is more receptive to the social context of information. Many doctors are alarmed that their patients do not understand what they are told: 'During the consultation, we explain everything to the patients! We ask them if they have understood and they say "yes". We get the impression that patients have understood when they leave the consulting room because we have explained everything and we ask if they have any questions and they don't.

---

12   This idea is often evoked in the medical literature, as Christine Delaporte's (2001) work shows. She believes that 'before announcing a diagnosis, the doctor should *feel* what the patient wants and what he/she is capable of taking in'.

13   I will give some examples further on of doctors badly interpreting patient's wishes, either in terms of information or therapy.

Ten days later, when an intern sees them again and asks them if everything has been explained, they answer: "No, no-one told me anything"! It is frustrating', said one oncologist. This oncologist was one of the doctors I was able to observe in consultations during which it was very apparent that the information he gave did not always answer the patients' questions (I will come back to this point). Some doctors justify not giving patients genuine information on their diagnosis by their incapacity to understand it and only provide this information to patients they presume to have sufficient understanding: 'We tell patients things depending on the understanding they have'. However, here too, it is necessary to question how the doctors are able to objectify both the capacity a person has to understand and the actual understanding they have of what they have been told. 'We can feel it', they explain. This again is a subjective, psychological judgement.

Frequently, doctors decide that patients are not able to receive certain pieces of information, such as their health status when it is too worrying, without realising that 30 years ago a doctor would have considered them unable to receive information that today they are given systematically. Justifying not informing a patient because of their 'psychological incapacity' of receiving the information shows that the doctors individualise and personalise the problem. This demonstrates that, at no point, is the problem perceived as a collective phenomenon partly resulting from a social and structural reality — that of the social treatment of the issue of information, linked to the historic condition of doctor–patient relationships. 'The doctor always gives information. The problem lies in managing patients' distress', said one oncologist. Beyond disagreements on the modalities of disclosure and on the best way of responding to patients' distress, everyone is in fact agreed in thinking that the problems are exclusively caused by the patient's difficulty to accept their illness; none think to question the quality of the information provided, nor indeed the reality of this information. The problem is psychologised, and at the same time it is de-sociologised. Yet the relational issues are not only psychological, we will see that they are also social, not only within the doctor–patient relationship but also between various health professionals, as shown by the demands of psychologists and nurses concerning their role in announcing an illness.

The same doctors also justify their decision to not inform patients of their health status by the risk they may be exposed to if they find out the truth and by the concurrent risk that they may commit suicide, a true leitmotif: 'They could throw themselves under a train if we tell them the truth. They will be traumatised. It is easy to make a law, but it is another whole thing to implement it!' The idea that the law on Patient Rights of 4 March 2002 is inapplicable relies on this fantasy that informed patients might commit suicide. Yet, it is interesting to note that, among all the doctors questioned on this point, none of them had had a case of an informed patient committing suicide, and that they never heard an example of such a situation. Sissela Bok (1984) also noted this, and wrote that it is very rare for a patient to commit suicide after being informed of a serious prognosis. But she added: 'And if they do, is it such an unreasonable reaction, and so against their own interests?' – a question that has to be placed in the context of the plea for truth that her work constitutes.

The prognostic dimension of diagnosis

There is evidently a large degree of imprecision in the phrase 'informing patients of their illness'. This phrase is commonly used in reference to the disclosure of a cancer which is why all doctors today claim to 'give the diagnosis', in line with the law obliging them to do so. Much has already been written about the debate on revealing a cancer diagnosis. We know that disclosure is considered cruel or inhumane in some countries where the diagnosis is systematically concealed, or just implied, while in other countries open and full disclosure is common practice. This second viewpoint is widely held in the United States where full 'disclosure' has become the norm, a result of the combined effect of social pressure, patient associations, legislation on informed consent and an increase in questioning of medical authority. The differing positions in different countries have not come about by chance, in that, as various works have shown, doctor-patient interactions are embedded in their cultural context and constrained by the contemporary cultural norms of the society they exist in. This relativist viewpoint is notably demonstrated by Holland et al. (1987).

However, whether the authors appeal for truth or for dissimulation, the debate generally overlooks the fact that, on one hand, pathological situations are mainly distinguished in terms of their seriousness, and on the other, cancerous disease has plural connotations today when, in the past, it had the single connotation as a lethal disease. Thus we cannot discuss the meaning of cancer in one society or another without taking into account its historical and dynamic character. Equally, we cannot claim that, these days, a cancer diagnosis is always disclosed to families, without specifying the type of cancer in question nor, above all, the degree of seriousness. Indeed, this aspect makes a fundamental difference.

So, what precisely is under discussion? And what diagnosis is really in question? In fact, while the presence of cancer may no longer be hidden, another reality many doctors now conceal is the presence of metastases. There is often silence surrounding this word, which has taken the fear-inducing image that the word 'cancer' used to have.[14] The current legal context, which prohibits the

---

14   Although as some doctors admit, the word is still sometimes difficult to say. 'I find it hard to say the word "cancer"', admitted one surgeon who has a reputation for sensitivity with patients. In his eyes, the word is still very violent: 'patients take it full in the face'.

reality of a patient's health status from being withheld, is not only linked to the struggles led by patient associations, but also to medical advances and to the increase in recovery rates. If doctors now more readily tell patients that they have cancer, it is because it is now considered to be more a chronic illness than a fatal one. But, on the other hand, doctors are much less willing to disclose the presence of metastases in the body because they have taken over the status cancer used to have. Thus, in the eyes of the actors at least, it is not rare for the diagnosis itself to already contain the prognosis. Telling patients 'your cancer has metastasised' provides them with information on both the nature of their affliction and on its possible progression, considering the fact that the diagnosis itself can signify a detrimental development. This is a case of what can be called the *prognostic dimension of diagnosis*. There has been a shift in the dissimulation that occurs today, in the 'not said'. The taboo has simply been moved to focus on a new object – another stage of the disease. From silence surrounding the illness itself, we have now moved to silence on its complication or aggravation, that is to say, on a diagnosis which, in the eyes of the actors, carries an implied prognosis.

Sharing information

Although, as we have seen, doctors generally agree with the doctrine that says precise information can only be given to patients on the condition that they want to know, but also that they should be able to both understand and accept the information, we will see that in reality, in a great number of cases, the basis of the criteria for whether patients should be informed or not is largely social. Observation of the consultation process revealed that the practice of only providing information on the development of their illness to patients who appear capable of 'taking the blow' (to cite the term that is often used) is very much present today. This capacity is at the very least inferred from the impression given by patients as to their psychological soundness, which is nevertheless relative and assessed by the doctor alone.

In fact, beyond the judgement made on the psychological ability of patients to receive precise and detailed information concerning their health status and the treatments proposed to them, this information is actually mainly given to people belonging to higher social categories, either because their distinction (in Bourdieu's sense of the term) leads to the assumption that they are better able to understand it, or because it engenders the assumption that they have a greater capacity to tolerate what is disclosed to them. The prognosis is even more likely to be only announced to someone who appears capable of hearing it. Mr R is a 66-year-old business manager who exudes confidence, he said:

My last scan was really bad, the nodules have grown very big. The doctor was very clear.
There is a new treatment based on antibodies that he wants to try but it will have to be

done with massive injections of Campto.[15] And so he has put me back on Campto. 'If that doesn't work, expect to move on sometime between now and 2004', he told me. Well, he didn't say it like that in fact but that is what he meant. Then the intern also told me that I didn't have long left. He said: 'The symptoms may well come back. If it doesn't work, they will come back in 6 to 12 months'. That clearly means that the organs have been affected and they can't guarantee they will function anymore, so after that, I'll have maybe 3 months left, no more. It was the intern who told me and it was confirmed by my doctor.

(It must be noted that following the provision of this information which is noticeably harsh, the patient's morale was badly affected and his oncologist had to prescribe psychoactive drugs.) Later, the patient explained:

This 6th molecule was important for me! And it worked well, the scan is excellent, the nodule is diminishing. The doctor gave me the choice: 'I could put you on stand-by, but it would be good to add a second layer'. I said 'OK'. Every other week until April. Today I am still going on 30km hikes. I have no exterior symptoms except during the three days when they stick the pump on me. I am beginning the 9th course of treatment and the markers are at 53,[16] it's almost normal! I know that even if my nodules are smaller now, they could start growing again in 6 months! I don't know much more but I don't ask the doctors. Anyhow, I know it won't change anything if I ask, so I try to bother people as little as possible.

Here, the patient experienced the disclosure of the possibility of a bad prognosis in a rather abrupt manner, when nothing was in fact certain. However, he had not actually asked any questions. The information was given to him because of the confidence he displays.

Information concerning the risks of a treatment is also more willingly given to patients with a socio-cultural level deemed to be compatible. Mrs A suffers from inflammatory polyarthritis, linked to rheumatoid scleroderma. Although she was satisfied with her care on a therapeutic level, she was not happy because her questions were not being answered and she lacked explanations on her affliction. She decided to consult a different doctor who explained:

With scleroderma, there is a risk of visceral involvement which could affect the lungs, the heart or the digestive tract, and there may be joint pain. The immune system is made to get rid of exterior agents (microbes, bacteria) but when the system is not working properly, it is either weakened (as in AIDS) or otherwise it becomes overactive (this is

---

15 Campto is generally used in treating advanced colorectal cancers. In some cases, it is associated with 5-fluorouracile (5FU), another anti-cancer agent.

16 The markers, measured in the blood, are an indication of tumoral activity.

case for allergies and auto-immune diseases). It can attack any organ and so it is treated with immunosuppressants (such as cortisone) but not too many, since if the immune system is too weak and we hit too hard, infections can result.

Later, in her absence, her doctor told me:

> That is enough of an explanation for patients. The treatment poses risks to the kidneys. Sometimes I conceal the side-effects of these medicines, for example methotrexate can cause pulmonary fibrosis and with Endoxan there is a risk of leukaemia – problems can occur 30 years later. But with this patient, I told her this since she has a sufficient cultural standing.

Consequently, it cannot be asserted that the differences between patients are only a function of their desire to know or of social determinants. It must be acknowledged that, as the field observations demonstrate, information is differently given depending on the patient's socio-cultural background.

In contrast to the inequalities in medical information that exist between industrialised countries and developing countries, Hoerni (1985) thinks there is a uniform exposure to medical information in our societies. He nevertheless observed that this information is differently received depending on the patients' cultural, educational and socioeconomic level. Although socially privileged and better educated patients ask more questions and express their points of view more than others, and, for this reason, are more likely to receive information (Street 1992), it is however noticeable that doctors pre-empt patient's questions or prejudge them according to their social background, thus demonstrating their social prejudice when evaluating the patients' information requirements.

Hooper et al. (1982) suggested that socioeconomic status affects the manner in which patients are treated on a therapeutic level. They showed that the higher their status, the more likely patients are to be seen by a doctor rather than a nurse, the more consultations they have and the more likely they are to undergo an intervention. They also showed that doctors give more information to older Anglo-American women than to younger Spanish-American men. This work is interesting in that it demonstrates the fact that patient characteristics affect doctor behaviour. But, in this study, the quality of information doctors provide is only correlated to ethnic origin, age or sex. My research shows that social affiliation and sociocultural level are much more determinant.[17]

---

17 The authors, who claimed that women receive better care, backed up their assertions by evoking the fact that they are more readily sent to a psychiatrist than men are for the same neurotic symptom. Such an analysis overlooks the invariable social fact that the social representation of women generally portrays them as more psychologically fragile, and more liable to be psychiatrised (Fainzang 1996).

Although observation of consultations clearly revealed that doctors tend to preferentially inform members of higher social classes, the doctors themselves do not appear to be aware of the influence of patients' social standing on the judgements they make concerning patient capacity to receive information. One business manager, with a degree from a prestigious business school, was given a very detailed explanation of the antibody-based treatments he was being proposed in order to strengthen his body's immune system. Although he had not explicitly requested the details because he knows doctors are very busy ('During the consultation, it is difficult, they don't have time, we can't stop them working!' he explained), the doctor gave him very precise information, based on the impression that he was able to understand because of his social bearing.

The same phenomenon can be seen in the case of a patient who was a teacher. 'My GP sent me to an oncologist', she explained. 'The other day, they were speaking on the telephone in front of me. I listened to what they were saying to try and find out more. I heard my doctor telling the other one, "go ahead, she's a teacher". I understood that the oncologist was asking if he should tell me the truth'. Another doctor, questioned after a consultation on the reasons he had informed a patient of her bad diagnosis so precisely, answered: 'She understands things well, I can tell her everything'. Yet another doctor said about a patient: 'It is obvious he has a high level intellectual profile'.

These observations must be cross-matched with the fact that doctors choose to withhold information from patients because 'they didn't ask me anything, and so they don't really want to know'. Not only are the doctors disregarding an important dimension which is that many patients, especially those from working class backgrounds, say they 'dare not ask' and so they are involuntarily reduced to ignorance on their own case because they do not know how to formulate the right questions or do not allow themselves to ask the doctors, but they also tend to assume patients want information, even when they do not formulate questions, when they think the patients are equipped with adequate cultural capital.

There are many examples that demonstrate how doctors more willingly impart a diagnosis or a type of treatment and its side-effects to patients according to their known or supposed social background, and to their, also presumed, cultural capital. Mr R, a 61-year-old chemical engineer, provides another example of a patient from a socioprofessional environment that makes it appropriate for the doctor to 'tell':

I had blood in my urine and a very sharp pain in the hip joint. My GP gave me an anti-inflammatory which relieved the pain but the bleeding continued. He sent me for an ultrasound of the bladder and they found a very large polyp in there. They operated on me and discovered that it was malignant (the surgeon told me after the operation). They couldn't take it all out, and they had to operate again a month later. He told me clearly, 'you also have metastases' and he sent me here for a general treatment because he couldn't just rely on a local treatment on the bladder. There were metastases in my lungs and bones.

A remarkable point on this subject is that doctors either base their judgement on detailed knowledge of the patient's files and the information concerning them (marital status, profession), or − when they do not have time to look at the whole file and they do not know the patient − on an impression given by the patient of their social standing.

Finally, although many doctors justify not providing information or not telling the truth by psychologising the problem and judging patients to be incapable of receiving it, the problem should also be addressed in social terms, taking into account the social mechanisms that govern the distribution of information. We have seen that, in fact, doctors' behaviour is regulated not only according to patients' psychological dispositions, but also very often according to their social characteristics which serve as the foundation of the judgment on the former. Added to the sadly well-known social inequalities in patient access to healthcare, is thus a *social inequality in access to information* furthered by this mechanism.

Around the Doctor

What role do other members of the healthcare team play?[18] In order to answer this question, it is necessary to contrast the perception patients have of the roles of various carers in distributing information concerning them with the perception the latter have of their role in information provision.

Patients almost unanimously observe a large disparity in the discourses of the different healthcare professionals caring for them in terms of their respective roles and their attitudes towards the obligation to inform patients. Mr G is 80 years old and has cancer of the prostate and colon. His wife is very angry about how little information the doctors are willing to impart concerning her husband's health status: 'They lied to my husband about his illness. I got angry again with Dr Z. He doesn't answer my questions. Dr R told me before his operation: "We won't pretend that there are no risks to this colon operation, because your husband is overweight and elderly". But Dr Z won't say anything'. Others question the different pieces of information they are given which are

---

18 The term 'healthcare team' should be considered in its broadest sense, in that it includes all the people who play a role in patient care, in one way or another (other specialist doctors, oncologists, surgeons, radiologists, interns, psychologists, nursing staff, clinical research associates, x-ray technicians), whether they are members of the team or not.

often incomplete. One patient complained that the doctors within one team do not always say the same thing, and that nothing is really explained to the patient: 'We are left in ignorance when we are the most concerned. This morning, they told me a third different version! It's unacceptable!'

Therefore, patients often choose to compare the discourses of different healthcare providers to assess the truth of their words, feeling satisfaction and relief when one person's words are confirmed by another. Others sometimes try to find out from one team member (notably interns) what they could not discover from their oncologist: 'The radiologist told me that there was a cyst, he did, you know, the iron thing … oh yes, it was an ultrasound. Dr I won't say anything at all, he won't take any responsibility! But with the poor intern, I insisted on knowing and he finally told me: "You have metastases measuring 11mm"!!' In this case it was the intern who revealed what the doctor wanted to conceal.

The existence of heterogeneous discourses within the medical team tends to instil a certain mistrust in patients who see this as a sign that something is being hidden from them. 'The doctor told me that it had all gone, that everything was fine, and this was just a preventative chemotherapy. But then a nurse told me: "It must be because there is something suspicious there"'. Patients are particularly sensitive to the existence of a contradiction between what two healthcare providers tell them, leading them to think something is being concealed, or that they are being lied to.

Patients thus often denounce the lack of coordination between healthcare providers. One patient's wife said: 'I told Dr H yesterday that the cardiologist had changed my husband's heart treatment. I know that the chemotherapy can be too strong for patients with heart problems; there is a risk. And since the cardiologist doesn't know anything about chemotherapy, I discussed this with Dr H. I told him that my husband had serious hypertension and asked him if there was any possible link with the chemotherapy. He answered: "Go and see your cardiologist, each to his own job"!' The patient's wife condemns what she called a 'medical gap' between different specialities which worries her greatly. Communication is not just thought to be lacking between doctors and patients but also between health professionals themselves.

From this point of view, many patients deplore the poor standard of information provision within the medical body itself. Mrs C is 58 years old and works as a cleaner at an old people's home; she has been under observation for 20 years for a cyst. She had a mammography and an ultrasound but the mammogram was negative (in fact it was a 'false negative'[19]), but the ultrasound revealed the presence of a nodule. She then underwent a biopsy but the cyst

---

19 Meaning that the results were wrongly deemed negative since she did in fact have a cancerous pathology which was found by the ultrasound.

tested negative after it was punctured. However, although the biopsy was negative, an MRI scan was requested and the results of this were 'suspect'. Finally, the patient underwent an operation to remove the nodule and ganglions as well as having a mastectomy. She was outraged: 'I have done so many tests, I don't understand why they haven't seen anything! I could understand it with people who don't have the tests, but not for me! My gynaecologist told me: "Everything is OK". Was she badly informed by the hospital services? She hadn't received the results of the breast tissue samples!' The patient doubts the effectiveness of communication and information sharing between professionals since she thinks that the hospital had not informed her GP. 'When I came back here, the doctor told me: "Oh, no! That is not right at all, this breast must be removed!" In fact, my gynaecologist had not received all the results, they had just told her that I had to see the doctor again'.

This lack of communication between healthcare providers is sometimes blamed on bad coordination, or sometimes on other reasons. Some also deplore the fact that financial interests influence therapeutic matters and that information is not communicated within the medical body itself:

> The surgeon from the clinic in T was furious that my husband was operated on here because he had done all the investigations at T. He said: 'I'm not going to serve it all to the hospital on a silver platter!' The colonoscopy showed the presence of a tumour, and he kept the report for 10 days before the hospital was informed! It was an emergency, but I am sure he wanted to create an emergency, an occlusion so that he would be able to operate on him at the clinic! I thought of lodging a complaint and I would have done if the operation had failed.

(The operation was a success. The complaint was thus not made but simply discussed with the anthropologist.)

Patients find it easier to ask for information from other healthcare providers than from the cancer specialist dealing with their case, especially if the specialist is a professor. They are convinced that they should not take up the doctor's valuable time by asking questions. They often ask a nurse, who is not always able to answer such questions. For example, a doctor left the room for a moment directly after having announced to his patient his proposal for a new treatment using antibodies in parallel to the treatment she had received previously. The patient then questioned the nurse: 'What is this new product he is talking about?' (He was talking about antibodies.) But the nurse did not answer on the subject of antibodies; her answer was related to the chemotherapy he had already had: 'I don't know which one he wants you to do again. You have had Campto and 5FU, but I don't know which one he wants to give you. It would be better to do the chemotherapy here'. The patient did not receive an answer to his question. When the doctor returned, he said: 'OK, we'll do that, shall we?'

But the patient did not answer. Later, when I saw him again, he complained that he had not received the information he wanted since the nurse had not answered his question.

Some people say they feel more at ease questioning the nursing staff than the doctors because their different status in the hospital hierarchy renders them more accessible. Contrarily, others prefer to ask their questions to the doctors, considering them to be more competent. Some patients target different people with their questions depending on the nature of the information required or the availability of the person being asked. One patient, a secretary, felt that: 'The laboratory technician explains the molecules and all that really well; we need more of these types of people, they have more time!'

Patients have no means of ascertaining the accuracy of the various pieces of information they receive. One of the problems is not so much whether information should be provided to patients or not because of the potential harm it could do, but that of the circulation of false ideas that take the status of information in patients' eyes because of the informer's professional status. This 'information' is not inconsequential and can sometimes do real harm, even when these consequences are social rather than therapeutic. Mrs A is a 58-year-old piano teacher with breast cancer. She questioned the hospital nurses about this disease. One nurse told her: 'Today we know that there is a link between breast cancer and psychological shocks experienced in relation to one's mother'. From that point on, the patient was convinced that this was the cause of her cancer and her relationship with her mother subsequently deteriorated.

Conversely, sometimes the nursing staff try to compensate for the harmful words of doctors. One patient, in the presence of a nurse who was preparing his intravenous drip, said: 'I am very well informed. There are many different treatments. I know there are some patients who have Ciplatine but I am getting Elvorine. There is also Campto. And that one really is the Rolls Royce! Some people get the Rolls Royces, for others it's the 2CV. I have the 2CV'. The nurse looked aghast and said: 'I didn't tell you that!!' He replied: 'No, it was the doctor!'

It is not necessarily easy for doctors to coordinate on the matter of patient information since there are many different approaches resulting from discrepancies in behaviour and options among healthcare providers. Between those who promote frank and total information and those who reveal nothing that could alarm patients, a whole range of attitudes are represented. And indeed, every doctor has an opinion on the behaviour of others: 'N is very harsh and unpredictable, he doesn't respect women; he palpates their breasts and then leaves them exposed while he talks to someone else'. 'D is very nice, he has a good rapport with his patients; he even gives them his phone number'. 'J is very comforting, too much so sometimes because it can then be difficult to put things right after him!' These quotes show that if the reality of information provision is partly a matter of personalities, this is just as much the case for those giving it as for those receiving it.

Some doctors prefer to let the radiologists inform their patients because of a tacit division of therapeutic work according to which radiologists should provide the diagnosis and oncologists the therapy. This does not correspond to what the patients say — they find that radiologists often offload the role to doctors. In fact, sometimes the radiologists do disclose the diagnosis, while in other cases they refuse to do so and send the patient back to their doctor. In reality, the difference in radiologists' attitudes partly depends on the context in which the radiological examinations are carried out. In the private sector patients are considered to be clients, so the examination results belong to them. Thus radiologists provide the information more readily and patients often leave with their results. On the other hand, in examinations carried out in the public sector or in non-profit private establishments, patients do not have direct access to the results. The documents must be given to patients during a consultation or interview, and the results can only be accessed if certain procedures are followed — often the patient must address a written demand to the head of the establishment.

What about the information provided by paramedical staff (nurses, supervisors, x-ray technicians)? These people are not authorised to answer patients' questions concerning test results or diagnoses. They can only provide information about treatments, their risks, effects and modalities. However, patients very often question them and they find themselves having to find ways of not revealing what they know or see.

Like oncologists, the majority of members of the healthcare team create a doctrine on the issue of information and on the role they are supposed to play in relation to their status and their place in the chain of actors caring for patients. For example, this nurse supervisor revealed the role she plays in the patient information process: 'The patients ask me questions to clarify what the doctor has said. When they leave the consultation, they ask me to say it all again. First, I ask them what the doctor told them'. The nurse supervisor wants to stay within the range of information given by the doctor and avoid saying too much. What she says depends on what the doctor has already divulged since he alone has the right to say or not say. She is given a document detailing the diagnosis, the examinations to be done and the procedure to be followed. 'Once', she said, 'I called a patient to tell him he was to go to hospital on a certain day for a treatment. He asked me: "What treatment? I didn't know about it!" There I realised I had gone too quickly. I told him that the doctor would call him to explain. In fact, I was relying on the document I was given, but he hadn't received the information at that point!' Another nurse said: 'What the patients want to know is how long it will last, how it is likely to go and if it will hurt. They don't generally ask us questions about the diagnosis. They don't ask the same questions to nurses as to doctors'. This point of view differs from that of another nurse who says patients turn to her when they have not received answers to the questions they have asked or would like to have asked the doctor, although she is aware of the limits of what she can say: 'When they want to know more about the diagnosis, I tell them to ask the doctor'.

A clinical research associate visits patients to assess the effects of trials – what are known as the 'responses' (resistance, side-effects) of the trial. Patients often take advantage of these visits to try and find out more, especially to ask them about the results of their tests. This associate has established a doctrine too, having found herself in an embarrassing situation on many occasions: 'At the beginning, if the results were good, I would tell them, but then if they turned bad afterwards, I didn't want to have to say. And so now, I don't say anything at all'.

Just as healthcare providers decide on the conditions and circumstances in which they give information or not, they may choose the conditions in which they decide to lie, or at least, become complicit in a doctor's lie. An oncologist's medical secretary regularly receives telephone calls from patients wanting to know more or have their test results. 'But I am not allowed to say. I tell them that I don't have them if the results are positive or that they will have to discuss it with the doctor; I am obliged to lie. But I tell them they don't have anything if the results are negative to stop them worrying for no reason'.

One nurse believes he is asked for information more frequently than doctors: 'We get all the questions on what will happen next – the prognosis, the treatment, the procedure, how many cures there are, whether people survive, and so on'. In reality it is very difficult to objectify such things considering the prestige professionals gain from being asked information, which pushes them into claiming a central role in the process. Nurses, in particular, have a tendency to lay claim to a position which puts them on a symbolic par with doctors and adds value to their social position. This aspect was especially obvious in staff meetings where everyone said they were particularly called upon on this subject but where the nurses were by far the most demanding: 'Nurses should be there to give information on the disease. Their role in the announcement procedure should be re-examined', one nurse said.

One of the most striking aspects is that the nurses act as spokespeople for the doctors. They internalise and echo doctors' convictions on information and become their ambassadors. This role is all the more gratifying and valorising since it allows them to be socially identified with the doctors. In particular, their discourses relate to patients' refusal to know, patients' denial, and the illusion of information. The nurses justify taking precautions with patients in terms of information thus: 'There are patients who say: "Go on, I am capable of hearing it all", who then break down. But if they ask us, we don't always know! If they are asking people who don't have the answers, it is because they don't really want to know!' Some nurses thus use the same type of psychologised reasoning in their recourse to interpretations such as 'denial'. Following the example of doctors – who are in turn greatly influenced by discourses created by psychologists – nurses analyse the fact that patients turn to them, obscuring not only the reality that patients do not necessarily know *who* within the medical team knows or does not know, and *who* is or is not in a position to inform them, but also the fact that it is easier for them to speak to a nurse than to a doctor, let alone to a 'professor'. Just as they overlook the power relations that prevail within the doctor–patient relationship, they overlook the power relationships that exist within a couple. One nurse said: 'When patients come with their spouse who speaks for them it means that they themselves do not want to know'. This somewhat quick conclusion demonstrates the difficulty nursing staff have in analysing patient behaviour other than by using a psychological reading of the 'refusal to know' type, and thus, their difficulty in examining the situation with the tools of sociological or anthropological analysis.

Likewise, the idea that nowadays patient information is provided in its totality is also shared and repeated by the nursing staff. 'Anyhow, in this department, we tell them everything!' one nurse claimed with satisfaction, demonstrating the medical staff's collective illusion surrounding the provision of information. Another said: 'I remember that 30 years ago we didn't say the same things. Instead of "we are going to operate", we said: "we are going to cure you", and instead of "we are going to give you chemotherapy", we said: "we are going to use an antibiotic therapy". We used to lie. But now we say everything'. A third nurse added: 'The patients know everything today. Their doctor tells them everything. As a matter of fact, people don't ask for further information. They know a lot, they know the protocols and they sign a consent form. If people don't ask anything, it is because they don't need to know and neither do they want to'. Added to the conviction that patients know everything, is the idea that when they don't know, they don't actually want to – as mentioned above. Equally the idea prevails that patients are 'fully informed' by their signature of consent. Further on, we will examine the reality of this consent and patients' perceptions of the information they gain from it.

Psychologists however hold a separate status within the healthcare team. Patients very rarely ask them for information. At most, they confide that they would like to know, or to be treated with more consideration. But their relationships with this professional are sometimes complex. As mentioned in the introduction, some patients want to talk about problems which they believe to be linked to the healthcare structure and methods of care provision but which have nothing to do with their own psychological state: 'They send us a psychologist when we complain'. Others refuse psychological care because they do not think that the need for dialogue is linked to a personal, psychological difficulty. In their eyes, the difficulty is inherent in the disease but exterior to themselves: 'We didn't want to talk to a psychologist. We told her we didn't want to. They act as if it was us with the problem, but the real problem is this disease that has hit us' (a patient, accompanied by her husband).[20]

When patients refer to a structural problem linked to the nature of doctor–patient relationships, psychologists often answer by detailing the difficulties doctors face. This follows a mechanism, once again, of personalising the phenomenon of information retention. Often, psychologists explain to patients that a doctor's refusal to inform them of the seriousness of a disease should be understood in terms of the doctor's own denial of death: 'The doctors reject the word "cancer" because it makes them uneasy, it is a way of refusing to confront it'. This is a typical psychological explanation, used to justify the doctors' failure to inform their patients of the reality of cancer – an explanation which, incidentally, does not take into account the fact that this information is unequally delivered according to the social background of the patient.

Doctors and Lies

The prevalent assertion, widely conveyed by health professionals themselves, that nowadays the truth is always told and information is always provided means they totally reject the existence of lying, a variation of under-information, or at the very least, claim that all deceptive practices have disappeared today. Hoerni (2005) wrote on this subject: 'We have gone from absolute paternalism to a point where the value of patient autonomy is entirely accepted. The time has now come to announce the demise of medical lies'. Equally, in allusion to a phrase written by J. Hamburger in a booklet entitled *Advice to Medical Students in my Hospital Department*, in 1963: 'One should lie in every case, without exception', Abiven (1996) commented that 'by asserting the necessity of lying in medical practice, J. Hamburger is only lending his authority to the most common practice of his time'. But has this practice really been abolished in our times?

Lies are just as much the dissimulation of one discourse as the production of another. We should be aware of the difficulty of distinguishing between a situation in which something is not said so as not to reveal it and a situation in which something is not said in order to make someone believe the opposite.[21]

---

20   It is worth noting that in a meeting, a psychologist lamented the fact that patient usage of the psychological support phone line was very low.

21   Although it also relies on Hippocrates' notion of decorum, on which the principle of beneficence is founded, this situation is totally distinct from that which Y. Jaffré (2002) described concerning the behaviour of healthcare providers in Mali, which consists of 'discursive avoidance' linked to the fact that it is not considered good to tell the truth since stating it is thought to imply that the enunciator would like it to happen.

When discussing lying, we are not simply referring to the well-known idea of 'lying by omission', commonplace in publications on the issue of truth in the medical domain, which can be more closely identified with 'silence' – although the boundary between one and the other is very porous. This research reveals the existence and the recognition of various types of lie, and it also shows the variability of the relationships between healthcare providers and lying depending on the place they occupy in the patient's care programme.

Actors qualify a statement as a lie without this always being an established fact. Thus, patients can receive information they believe to be true when it is in fact false, but conversely, they can receive information they believe to be false when it is in fact true. This is why the issue of lying will be examined here in all its different aspects: both as a suspected fact and as an established fact, on the part of the actors, without prejudging the awareness the person being duped does or does not possess. We will see, on one hand, that lying is not the preserve of doctors but that it is also part of the patients' behaviour, and on the other hand, that it is a weapon that is frequently employed since lying is an integral part of therapeutic relationships as it is of all social relationships.

The praise of lying

Doctor's lies are explained and justified in various ways. We can find some of the same models that explain and justify lying in those concerning the retention of information and the dissimulation of truth. A lie is simply one step further. It is also common to evoke the concept of 'humane lying', as illustrated by this oncologist: 'It's better to lie to them. Anyhow, they know the truth, I'm not going to make matters worse!' Psychologists however analyse doctor's lies as 'lying through weakness' in reference to the psychological reasons, such as the fear of death and the difficulty of facing up to the truth, that prevent them from telling the truth. Lying is thus interpreted as a 'defence mechanism' (see Ruszniewski 1995).[22] Here again, the same explanatory models are at work.

Some doctors justify their lies not by the fact that they are incapable of telling the truth, but because the patients are incapable of hearing it. To illustrate this incapacity in patients, a psychiatrist said: 'It is always difficult to hear it, that's for sure! There are no good ways of telling people they have cancer. It is like telling them they are being cheated on! The patients are furious when we tell them that! So if the doctor doesn't want to lose his clients, well, he won't say it, or he will say something else! He can't do otherwise!' Here, the doctors pass

---

22   In reference to the psychologists' explanation that doctors lie through weakness, Moley-Massol (2004) said about this defence mechanism used by healthcare providers that the stated objective for lying is to spare the patient but it is in fact to spare the doctor and occasionally the family from the patient's reaction.

insidiously from silence to lying, from the act of saying nothing to the act of saying 'something else', to such an extent that there is a shift from the idea of the difficulty of telling the truth to the idea of the inevitability, or even the necessity, of lying.

Finally, for others, telling lies is the lot some healthcare providers cannot escape because of the place they occupy in the health system or in the organisation of care. Dr L works in day hospital department, he believes he has an easier role than other doctors because 'the worst has already been done', he said, in reference to diagnostic disclosure. 'The patients already know what is wrong with them when they come here. They have already received the bad news in a consultation. It is the doctors holding consultations who have to make the announcement. It's just like the cops – there are the goodies and the baddies. We are the goodies, we reassure them afterwards. If people want explanations, they can ask us – we are there to support them after the consultation. We spend all our time lying, we lie all day to provide a little comfort!' This is how this doctor sees the division of tasks: doctors holding consultations are there to tell the truth while the day hospital doctors lie.

We have seen that doctors often only provide information to patients in order to fulfil their therapeutic objectives. Katz (1984) showed in reference to what he called 'altruistic silence' that information is only given in order to encourage patients to make a decision which conforms to their doctor's opinion. Yet, doctors often withhold information on the risks of a treatment and discourage patients from reading the information leaflets on pharmaceutical products (Fainzang 2001) with the aim of inciting them to follow their prescription. Moreover, they also choose to conceal the possible side-effects of the treatments and even try to mislead patients on this subject to avoid the risk of the information dissuading patients from taking the medicine prescribed. Some doctors will go as far as contradicting the information contained in the information leaflets, so that their patients accept the treatment. Thus there is a tendency among many doctors, not only to *withhold information* about the illness, its treatments, its reasons and its risks, but to *lie* to them, in particular by claiming the contents of the leaflets on the possible side-effects of medicines to be false in order to persuade patients to take them. The practice of lying is, in this respect, a regular component of the behaviour of the medical body. By contradicting the information provided by pharmaceutical laboratories on the possible side-effects of medicines as detailed in the leaflets, these doctors produce a deceptive discourse in order to achieve their objectives. Patients do not generally question this discourse. The aura of truth surrounding the medical discourse is linked to what Foucault (1980) named 'the political economy of truth', one characteristic of which is to take the form of scientific discourse (see Tambiah 1990).

Doctors sometimes justify their lies by claiming the truth to be useless. Useless truth is contrasted to useful information which, as we have seen, is often the only condition in which some doctors inform their patients. Multiple logics are thus invoked to account for lying.

The practice of lying is demonstrated by the doctor's own accounts, which the literature on the subject reflects. While they sometimes take refuge behind the claim that they are not lying but remaining silent (R. Brauman, the president of Médecins Sans Frontières, suggested the nuance: 'I don't lie, but I sometimes have to remain silent'.), or absolve themselves by evoking 'the attitude that consists not of lying, but avoiding the use of terms that induce fear' (see S. Merran, a scan radiologist, who said, 'there is a little thing on the lung'), they also sometimes admit to lying. S. Merran said: 'To be honest, we do sometimes tell barefaced lies', and D. Khayat, head of a medical oncology service admitted: 'We do sometimes lie. Yesterday, I lied to a patient with lung cancer with metastases' (see Favereau 1994: 24).

Finally, we can see that between dissimulation and lying, two practices that are nonetheless distinct, the difference lies more in the degree to which they are practiced than their nature. The negative labelling of the term 'lie' is however what makes people reluctant to use it to describe doctors' behaviour[23] and the addition of 'by omission' generally intends to exonerate the liar.

On the whole, doctor's lies are justified by a rationalising discourse which lends them legitimacy. Many studies agree in morally justifying doctors' lies by evoking patients' refusal to know (or refusal of the truth for those who fear it) or because of the harm the truth could do. Plato wrote in *La République* that only doctors and chiefs of cities possessed the right to lie, the former in the interest of their patients and the latter in the interest of the city.[24] Thus, in all cases, justifications are made for doctors' lies. Barnes (1994) purports the existence of 'permissible' lies and shows that the manuals on medical ethics often include a section on the lies that can be told to patients if they are dying, if they are receiving placebos or if they are taking part in clinical trials.

Equally, in his book *Réflexions sur le mensonge* (*Thoughts on Lying*), Alexandre Koyré summed up the main philosophical and moral points on the subject of lying thus: 'Although the positive and active forms of lying, *suggestio falsi*, are intransigent, they are much less so in their negative and passive state, *suppressio veri*. It is known that, as the proverb says, "some things are better left unsaid".

---

23   If this negative labelling is what the use of the term 'pious lying' aims to eliminate, it is striking to note nevertheless that it doesn't characterise the terms 'silence' or 'secret'. In many social situations, secrets are valorised whereas lies are devalorised: indeed, we often swear to keep a secret, but we never swear to tell a lie.

24   Even though he added later that 'for every other person, lying is forbidden, and we maintain that the individual who lies to a chief commits a fault of the same nature but more serious, as the patient who does not tell the truth to his doctor'.

At least they should not always be said. And not to everyone' (Alexandre Koyré 1996). This is another way of restoring 'lying by omission' to favour.

The specificity of medical lying, as opposed to the practice of lying in ordinary social life or in politics, has lead a significant number of authors to question the validity of qualifying it as a lie. This is notably the case for those who adopt a relativist perspective and refute the designation, believing that if it is not experienced as a lie, it is not a true lie. Armstrong (1987) took this type of approach, using a diachronic perspective to show that 'a lie only exists in a relationship to a regime of truth which enables it to be identified as such'. He reproached Aries (1982) for considering the retention of the prognosis of imminent death from the patient to be the lie that dominated the period between the mid-nineteenth and twentieth centuries. In Armstrong's view, rather than blaming this epoch for having been silent on the truth, it should be established whether what is now a lie in our eyes, was so at that time. He thinks that, in the process of transformation from one regime of truth to another, there exist several stages of which the first is to recognise whether silence can be constructed as a lie or not, thus highlighting that lying is a social and historical construction. This perspective is also adopted by other authors who argue, from a synchronic perspective, in accordance with the precepts of cultural relativism, that lies considered acceptable in one society are not considered so in another.

Alongside cultural relativism, a moral relativism has emerged which is not only illustrated by the position of some philosophers such as Jankélévitch (see Coll. 1966), who believes that only those who falsify the truth *in their own interests* lie,[25] but also, by those taking a sociological approach such as Schein (2004). In his investigation of the behavioural norms influencing information provision, Schein noted that lying is not in itself a moral issue. He believes that what makes it a moral issue is the degree to which the liar's intention is destructive and the degree to which the person being lied to is subjected to harm as a result of the lie. He recognises that learning to lie or withhold some versions of the truth is fundamental to the maintenance of social order. Schein thinks that the norms concerning what is moral or immoral change depending on the professional environment or professional community. Each professional community establishes norms that dictate what information can and cannot be told, and who can be lied to, on what subject, and what interests should be protected. He believes that the truth is 'defined by cultural norms', and that everyone follows the same rules, whether in marketing, development or

---

25 He thus defined a lie through its benefit for the liar. (We could argue that such a definition is not unproblematic since there is no certainty that the doctor is not benefitting by falsifying the truth, either in facilitating − at least from his point of view − his work in caring for the patient, or by avoiding the potential difficulty of telling the truth, or by reinforcing his position of dominance over the patient.)

research. However, it is not certain, as Stein claims, that there really exists such a homogeneity in the implementation of these norms in terms of lying and information. In the medical domain, the very controversy that exists between doctors on this issue shows that the rules are not always followed in the same way. By reducing the cultural to the professional, Schein ignores the fact that these norms come into contact with other norms, greatly complicating their role as a model.

Finally, the relativist perspectives (historical, cultural or moral) partly resemble Hacking's (1982) nominalist perspective. He adopted Hamlet's maxim on good and evil and transposing it to the issue of truth, he wrote: 'Nothing is either true or false, but thinking makes it so'.

A striking element of the debates on the ethical dimension of lying is that their justifications for recommending it or condemning it are almost always based on the interests of the person being lied to. The mechanism by which doctors' lies are based on ethics, is precisely that it relies on the idea that lies are told to the benefit of the person being lied to and not the liar, the opposite of what occurs in politics, where the archetypal thought in this respect is that of Machiavelli. The idea is that the liar gains no benefit from this deception. This vision results from the social image of doctors that has developed in our societies. This activity, however rational it may seem in the sense that there are therapeutic 'reasons' behind it, conveys the liar's adhesion to determined cultural patterns. But we will also see that as a social phenomenon, the practice conforms to social mechanisms which are not always consciously acknowledged by the actors. From this point of view, the ethical debate is anchored in utilitarian philosophy. For utilitarians, the justification of an act is determined by the positive or negative nature of its consequences. In utilitarian philosophy, the decision to lie is thus made after having assessed its risks or benefits. A doctor's lie thus typically falls under a utilitarian philosophy which gives it a legitimacy based on its consequences, its usefulness.

While justification for a doctor's lies is visible through the appellation '*pieux mensonge*' (pious lie) in French, which aims to strip the lie of any negative value, it is also found in the English term the 'noble lie' ('noble' because it is accomplished for a good cause). But, there too, some authors ask: Who can determine to what extent the cause is good? This is what Sissela Bok (1979) meant when, in her work of moral philosophy, she asked whether lying is ever harmless, even in the case of 'pious' lies. In the English-speaking world, a more sophisticated model has been developed, which makes a distinction for so-called ethical lies between *white lies* and *noble lies*. White lies are lies that aim to not cause harm and have low moral implication (Bok gave the example of telling someone they have a nice tie when it is in fact horrible, or telling a guest that the vase they have just broken is not valuable). White lies are lies in which nothing important is at stake (Nyberg 1993). However, according to Bok, the judgement on the harmlessness of a white lie is subjective, just as it is for a noble lie, and she denounces its use for this reason. She criticises utilitarianism by saying that what the liar perceives to be inoffensive or even beneficial to the person being lied to, cannot be so in the eyes of the latter. She also used the example of the placebo to show the danger inherent in this lie and the harmful effects concealed within it (loss of trust in the medicine and the doctor). Sissela Bok thus rejects the arguments doctors use to justify lying to patients by saying that the risks of telling the truth are less than they are thought to be and the benefits are higher. In so doing, she also takes a utilitarian perspective on truth. She remarked for example that patients follow instructions better when they know what their disease is and why they have been prescribed such a treatment.[26]

Even when they are medical, lies are sometimes condemned on an exclusively ethical basis, in line with Kant's position that all lies are immoral, whatever the reasons and circumstances, for the reason that once a law authorises lying in certain cases, nobody can believe anybody anymore. The judgement on the benefits of lying is thus subject to controversy. For his part, Durandin (1993) distinguished between two large categories of lies (those which serve the interests of the liar him/herself, and those, said to be charitable, that are told, in principle, in the interests of others). But, taking an opposing view to the authors who justify medical lying as 'pious lying', he put this distinction in perspective by declaring: 'When deciding to tell a pious lie, we are treating the person we lie to as a minor because we are assuming the right and the ability to make a judgement as much on their true interests as on their present level of understanding. Consequently, a pious lie, however well intentioned, creates a relationship that excludes equality'.

Lying can be considered within a specific social relationship, namely, within a power relationship. Lying is of course in itself an exercise of power and retention of knowledge since the doctor jealously guards the knowledge from the people dependant on him/her. Roqueplo (1974) showed that the retention of knowledge is a means to protect one's own place in the social hierarchy and that sharing knowledge also involves sharing power. Likewise, reducing the social distribution of knowledge through lying is a sociological mechanism that is well demonstrated by Gilsenan (1979), who showed that it is intricately linked to the system of power and control of any society. Indeed, the same logic is at work in very different societies. Among the Bissa of Burkina-Faso, the existing links between lying and truth on one side and power on the other are expressed through rules governing the diffusion of divinatory diagnoses.

---

26 'Not telling the truth is better for whom?' she asked, demonstrating the subjective nature of this judgement, and rejecting the idea that only powerful people can know what is good for others, and that those they deceive are incapable of making an appropriate judgement on the situation.

Thus, the divinatory consultation and the diffusion of its results obey a very precise codification that follows rules concerning access to knowledge. And the knowledge concerning diagnoses does not escape these rules. A younger man, who may be an adult, is obliged to tell the truth to his elders, but he has the right to lie to women (Fainzang 1986). Indeed, lying is an ingredient of political life, in that it is a weapon or strategy in the service of power.[27] The lies told by doctors may share certain characteristics with lies told by those who hold political power and in this sense they are a tool that serves medical power, but they are nevertheless specific in that they are still rationalised and legitimised, and even justified on ethical grounds.

Secrets, silences and lies

The notions of secrets, truth and lies inevitably play a role in how medical information is shared with patients. Indeed, the discourse of secrets or truth (more precisely, the difficulties inherent in telling the truth or the necessity of keeping a secret) is often employed in the accomplishment of the practice of lying. Focusing on the respective places occupied by secrets and lies in medical practice amounts to examining what lying and secrets have in common, in what ways they are different, and the conditions in which a secret becomes a lie.

The anthropologists who have investigated the issue of secrets have shown the links they have with power (Augé 1974; Zempléni 1976; Jamin 1977). These studies provided striking analyses in that they highlighted the power involved in the very fact of withholding information. The alliance between power and speech is a phenomenon that exists in social functioning in general. Social law is inseparable from the law of silence, according to which the strategy of power is to say nothing (Augé 1974). For Jamin (1977) too, the exercise of power can only be acquired or maintained by appropriating and retaining speech. He thinks that the links between secrets and power are objectivised by the fact that the importance of secrets lies less in what they hide than in what they reveal, that is, one's affiliation to a certain class or status.

While secrets are closely linked to silence, lies are just as much the dissimulation of one discourse as the production of another. In the medical domain, secrets take a different meaning depending on whether the person being lied to is a patient or not. Unlike medical confidentiality, where health professionals and patients may share the secret of a diagnosis, thus creating a link between the two parties, lying creates a distance between the actors. It does not unite doctor and patient in the face of others, it separates one from the other. However, a

---

27   On this point we can refer to Rabaté's (2005) work, a philosophical meditation on lying, and on lies in politics in particular. In this regard he used some elements of Koyré's (1996) thinking on the political function of modern lying.

secret very quickly becomes a lie once the patients are not told the truth about their own condition and are deceived as to their health status. Dumoulin (1981) said: 'Secrets are a means of command, allowing doctors to be obeyed in their prescriptions, by avoiding any discussion or by leading the conversation in a false direction. It allows doctors to tolerate a situation that would otherwise be intolerable – facing a challenge to their decisions or a relationship with a client living with a difficult situation'. We can doubtless discuss lying in the same terms. Lies are thus closely linked to secrets but they can however be decisively distinguished. Lies cannot be confused with secrets to the extent that, in a lie, there is a more active element. For Simmel (1991), not saying and lying are the passive and active forms of secret keeping.[28] Nonetheless, secrets and lies maintain links of reciprocal inclusion since a secret can imply a lie and a lie necessarily supposes a secret; in other words, it involves keeping the truth secret.

Close links therefore exist between secrets and lies. These are clearly demonstrated when they are seen as a means of exercising one's power or of controlling the behaviour of others. Indeed, when H. Arendt (1972) discussed secrets as a mean of control, she also included in this, 'deception, deliberate falsification and outright lies, used (by dominant parties) as a legitimate means of achieving their (political) objectives'.

Most healthcare providers, and particularly doctors, create for themselves a doctrine of lying which partly overlaps with their criteria for refusing information, but is more explicit. The criteria vary from one healthcare provider to another. They can include:

- The people being lied to: 'We lie more often to younger people; we tend to want to protect them more', one doctor confided.
- The type of diagnosis (lies are thus related to the degree of seriousness of the disease and particularly to the presence of metastases): '90 per cent of metastatic cancers are incurable and so telling them they have metastases is like telling them it is over! There is no point in giving destructive information if there is no benefit for treatment adherence', one oncologist said. (As discussed above, although cancer has become a chronic illness nowadays, and disclosure of such a diagnosis has become less alarming, the presence of metastases now has the status of an equivalent to a death sentence formerly occupied by cancer itself.)
- The type of treatment: 'If patients go from a curative treatment to palliative care, meaning they have no chance of recovery, I don't inform them. I tell them that we are treating them, but they don't know that it is a palliative treatment, an end of life treatment, simply prescribed to manage the pain since the anti-cancer treatment has been stopped. There is no point in telling them because

---

28   Petitat (1998) also provides a sociological study of secrets.

it has no bearing on the treatment. It's the type of treatment that makes me decide whether to tell the truth or not'. Another said: 'When we give them chemotherapy because it is not possible to operate, we can't explain to the patient that there is no point in operating because there are too many [metastases]; that is not possible'.

- The examination results: one radiologist pretends he cannot read the scan results immediately and leaves the oncologist the task of disclosing the results to patients.

Every doctor thus places the boundary between the sphere of truth and that of lies at a different stage or outcome. In this regard we can say there is variability both in the threshold and the register of the lies consciously told by doctors.

On rare occasions, doctors claim to lie when they believe the information to be unspeakable; for example, a problem related to healthcare politics.

[One patient is told she is at risk of a brain haemorrhage:]

The patient: Oh! That worries me! I don't want to turn into a vegetable! I'd rather go straight away!

The doctor: No! I am painting the darkest picture to convince you of the need to stay in hospital. But we don't have enough platelets. We can't give you a transfusion and we can't make the platelets either − there are not enough blood donors.

[The doctor told me however:]

If she has a brain haemorrhage today, her life will only be shortened by a few months, it won't be a tragedy. I didn't want to request platelets and I didn't ask the blood centre because I don't want to use platelets for her that could save a 20-year-old man's life. I told her that there weren't any but I instructed them not to order any.

Here, the lie concerns the availability of platelets. To tell her that he does not want to ask for them in her case would make clear the pointlessness of such a strategy in view of the seriousness of her disease.[29]

We have seen that doctors use all sorts of tricks and invent different techniques in order to euphemise the illness when they have to inform patients of their condition. This euphemisation sometimes leads them to give false information, and therefore, to lie. Patients sometimes expose this false information inducing doctors to try to reduce the amount of false content

---

29 We should note, as an epilogue, that the patient then asked her family, and one family member was willing to donate some blood for her.

by correcting it, and in doing so they produce a new lie. A doctor had told his patient that he had a polyp rather than cancer and the patient has just had an operation on the rectum:

The patient: I must say, you sent me for a big operation for just a polyp!

The doctor: It wasn't a polyp.

The patient: You mean it was cancer?

The doctor (embarrassed): It was a pre-cancerous lesion which would have become a cancer in a few weeks.

The doctor thus found a different phrase, which was a little closer to the truth, but was still a lie. He told me: 'That was more acceptable. In fact, it was a lie since the "pre" in pre-cancerous was false. He really did have cancer, but it allowed him to come to terms with his illness and treatment without being traumatised'.[30] We can see that, in order to compensate for a lie discovered by the patient, the doctor tells another which is closer to the truth but that is still not actually true. Lies can thus be told in stages.

In the same way that information is only given to people judged capable of receiving it, and that the truth is only told to people judged able to hear it, lies are only not told to those doctors judge capable of dealing with the truth. It seems the truth must be distilled, distributed like a treatment, following recommended doses and adapted to each patient. It is as if doctors are ensuring there are no negative side-effects. Somehow, lying is adopted as a therapeutic strategy in order to prevent an iatrogenic truth.

Lying can reside in a manipulation of the truth, through leading the patient to false conclusions. The doctor dealing with a young man suffering from Hodgkin's disease confided: 'In his case, there is a 50 per cent chance of surviving after five years. I wasn't going to tell him he will die within five years! So I told him: "There is a 50 per cent chance of complete recovery after five years". It was up to him to ask me what happens to the others! But he didn't ask …' The lie here relates to the presentation of the alternative, through the use of the expression 'complete recovery'. 'Complete recovery' has in fact

---

30 We could comment on this incident – but the commentary is peripheral to my point here – by saying that there is no certainty that the patient was not more disturbed to discover that the nature of his illness had been hidden from him by talking of a polyp, and by asking what he will now do with this information concerning the existence of a 'pre-cancerous lesion'. What trust does he have left in the doctor who he knows lied to him the first time? In this we can assess the perverse effects of such techniques in which doctors 'euphemise' the illness.

two possible antonyms, in relation to both the word 'recovery' and the word 'complete'. We should note the deceptive nature of the phrase in that it aims to make the patient believe that the alternative to recovery is not death but partial recovery. In doing this, the doctor is telling the truth, but it is a distorted truth.

Lying can also consist of a manipulation of terms or phrases whose ambiguity allows the doctor to make the patient believe something other than what he is really saying.

A doctor does not want to tell his patient, who is suffering from liver cancer, that his condition is serious and that his life is threatened. A significant decline in his platelets means he is at risk of an internal haemorrhage or a brain haemorrhage. The doctor tells him: 'We will be treating you like a crystal vase'.

The patient must have understood: 'We will treat you very well, very gently', whereas the doctor actually thinks he is as fragile and vulnerable as a crystal. The information which supposedly informs him of his health status is phrased in such a way that the patient understands it to be information on the quality of his care.

Mrs C has incurable liver cancer and her life expectancy is very short. The doctor told her they needed to take a 'therapeutic break', meaning that in reality her treatment had failed and it had to be stopped: 'We have abandoned any ambition of finding a cure. In fact, we have given up, but I prefer to tell her we are taking a break'.

Although doctors willingly and consciously define the conditions and criteria in which they lie, on the other hand, they are not necessarily aware that they are much less likely to lie to patients from more privileged sociocultural backgrounds. Just as information is only given, as seen above, to those thought to have the ability to understand it because they show signs of belonging to a higher social and cultural class, conversely, patients from less advantaged backgrounds are more often lied to. When discussing a farmer with lymphoma (cancer of the lymph glands), a medical oncologist said: 'We can cure him, he could easily live to 95, but it is better not to tell him he has cancer. We can't tell the truth to a patient whose cultural situation makes him incapable of receiving the information. For him, cancer means death. But in fact there would be a greater risk of him dying by throwing himself out of a window than from his cancer'.

Within the practice of lying, there is thus both an expression and a reinforcement of social differences in how patients are treated in terms of information.

Lying, as practiced by doctors, is thus linked to the specific position they occupy within the doctor–patient relationship and to the exercise of power that characterises this position. The exemplary realisation of this power is the appropriation of the patient's body. From this point of view, the choice doctors make as to whether to tell the truth or lie is only partially personal. Their behaviour is the result of a social construction, both of their role and their place in the doctor–patient relationship, which shapes them, models them and teaches them to lie. Doctor's use of lying is the result of a learned, socialised way of positioning oneself in the medical relationship.

In this attempt to provide an overarching view on the meaning, use and role of doctor's lies as regards their patients, it is noticeable that the use of lying is the result of two processes − that of rationalisation and that of cultural socialisation. Indeed, although lying is rationalised, its expression relies on a cultural logic under which doctors possess knowledge and power that authorise them to not tell the truth. The rationalisation presiding over this practice cannot by itself explain it since doctors' lies find anchorage in a cultural model of construction of the relationship of authority. Lies are thus driven by cultural reasons and symbolic logics, and not only by ethical or practical reasons. Besides, as we have seen, it is both for ethical and/or practical reasons that individuals choose to do one thing or its opposite: tell the truth or tell a lie.

Chapter 2
The Patients

Patients and Information

According to the research on the subject, there are many patients who want to be informed about their cancer and its development, and take an active role in their care programme (Degner and Sloan 1992; Blanchard et al. 1998; Charles et al. 1999), although their behaviour concerning the search for information is closely linked to sociodemographic factors (Beisecker and Beisecker 1990). Therefore we cannot discuss 'contemporary patients' without taking their social and cultural characteristics into account. However, these studies are all quantitative and do not show precisely how patients perceive the information they receive, the exact nature of their requests, but above all, how they behave in practice as regards information within the doctor–patient relationship. Moreover, the statistical studies aiming to discover the percentage of patients who want to obtain information are sometimes only of limited use since patients and doctors have a very different understanding of the term 'information', and of the phrase 'obtaining information'. I will cite for example the case of a patient who wanted to have all the information on her prognosis excepting technical information. She did not want to know the details of her illness because she did not want to 'visualise' it, but she wanted to know where she should place this illness in her life. Finally, the limitations of studies on the search for information carried out through questionnaires are revealed when we notice that, in the field, some patients claim to have asked for information when in reality they have not.

Gathering personal accounts, but also observing patient behaviour during consultations, provides insight into their experiences in terms of the information searched for and obtained or not in the hospital service they frequent and on their tangible behaviour in this domain (their expectations on the subject, the information they themselves give to doctors, the questions they ask or do not ask). Some of the themes addressed in the previous chapter on doctors will thus be examined here, in mirror image, to unravel where the perceptions and practices of each side are echoed and where they are contradicted. I will then discuss the role played by the patients' families in accessing information. Finally, I will approach the specific issue of lying on the part of the patients. To do this, I will not only examine the perception they have of the doctors' discourses, but also the practice of lying that they themselves partake in, in order to discover their mechanisms, symmetries and distinctive features.

Of course, patients' reactions are not homogenous, if only because individuals vary greatly and react differently in accordance with their own history and personal dispositions. The psychological dimension of the way information concerning a disease is managed cannot, of course, be ignored. Although I have questioned above the way doctors rely exclusively on this type of explanation to build their doctrine on information provision, this does not mean I ignore the importance and diversity of patients' psychological profiles. A patient suffering from thyroid cancer was told by her doctor: 'There is a 99 per cent chance of recovery in your case'. She replied: 'The 1 per cent will stop me from sleeping tonight!' This case perfectly illustrates the diversity of patient reactions since, in contrast, as the doctor himself said: 'Sometimes patients focus on a 10 per cent chance of recovery, and that helps them to sleep'.

Patients thus react very differently to information, not only in terms of their prospects of recovery and the percentages they are given, but also regarding the treatments proposed, in that the latter can be seen as an indicator of the seriousness of the diagnosis. Thus, some patients are overwhelmed when they discover they will undergo an operation, while others feel this way when they discover they will undergo chemotherapy. Mrs T said: 'I took my mastectomy well. The hardest thing was discovering I had to have chemotherapy. That really shocked me. It meant it was really serious'.

However, beyond the diversity of patient reactions attributable to the diversity of their psychological profiles, I will try to unearth the collective logics on which their attitudes are based in order to attempt to determine the way in which their status as patients influences their relationship with information.

Patients, whatever their social background and despite what the doctors believe, generally want to know as much as possible about their affliction − the exact nature of the diagnosis, the development of the disease, the possible treatments and their effects and risks − even though, as we will see, they do not always ask. Information is primarily perceived to be necessary, in a strictly therapeutic sense. The need to be informed is connected to the need to agree to the treatment proposed by the medical body, and for this, to understand what is at stake. There is no lack of examples of patients who try to refuse a treatment because they are not convinced of its necessity having been under-informed as to the seriousness of the situation. This type of information is sometimes the only one that counts in the patient's eyes. Mrs C (a bursar) said: 'I was given the information, the professor read it all out to me to convince me to have a mastectomy. I didn't understand any of it but it was just to make me understand that it had to be removed. I understood that it was serious'.

This echoes the practical dimension of information, on the grounds of which the doctors recommend informing patients. It is either a case of worrying patients enough for them to understand the seriousness of their condition and agree to the treatment proposed (whatever their degree of understanding of the illness itself), or to simply provide them with the elements of information necessary to encourage them to follow the treatment. After his consultation with the oncologist, Mr G (64 years old) said: 'I know the treatment seems to be working and I need to continue with the chemotherapy. That is all I know'. For these patients, the information given in consultation consists for the most part of divulging what is necessary for the treatment to be followed.

Contrary to what some doctors believe, the need to know cannot be reduced to the desire to hear only good news. The uncertainty in which the patients find themselves is often very distressing (see Ménoret 1999), much more it seems that knowing a diagnosis, or even a serious prognosis. Mr L is a head waiter, suffering from sarcoidosis and inflammation of the upper lobes in the lung and the ganglions between the lungs, with a risk of pulmonary fibrosis. He said:

> They took out a submaxillary ganglion, I have been through all the hospital departments. They analysed it and diagnosed the disease. There are two types – a quick one and a chronic one. But they don't know how it is caught, it seems. When I ask them, they say they don't know. And then they tell me: 'you will perhaps recover'. I don't like that. I don't know if it is because they don't want to tell me anything, or if they really don't know. I'd like to be sure. I would rather they said: 'No, there are no chances of recovery, but we will keep you as you are'.

Mr J (a 52-year-old computer specialist) knew that he had colon cancer with pulmonary metastases. However, he was not informed that his metastases had 'doubled' and that, despite the operations and multiple courses of chemotherapy:

> It grew back straight away somewhere else. They tested me every three months, but it was growing back. When it was too big, they took it out. They operated on me three times then gave me more chemotherapy. This one seems to be working – the metastases have stopped growing. They have got smaller with my current treatment (Campto). They took out two whole lobes of the lung. At the start, they concealed the fact that the metastases were growing from me. They told me: 'there are marks'. And so when they announced the need for an emergency operation, I didn't agree to it!

The discrepancy here between what is disclosed (the diagnosis) and recommended (therapy) is counterproductive. In the eyes of patients themselves, the doctors' tendency to hide the urgency of the situation has the effect of not making them ready to accept a treatment. A situation which patients are very aware of, sometimes after bearing the consequences: 'Since then, they don't lie anymore, they show me everything!' The situation is made even more difficult to manage in terms of care provision when there is also a discrepancy between the diagnosis announced and the symptoms the patients experience: 'They had to show me the scans. Otherwise I wouldn't agree to the operation, it was the size of an orange!! I couldn't feel anything, that's why I didn't want it!'

The patients' desire to know is also partly based on the conviction that they could usefully anticipate an aggravation of their disease – not by agreeing to a treatment, but by reacting to the illness in an appropriate manner. Mrs G, a 66-year-old teacher, said:

> After my operation, my goddaughter gave me a book by Dr Israël. I learnt a lot from this book. If I had known before the operation, I would be better by now! I learnt what R.0. is, 0 resection means there are no metastases on the liver – the markers are at 0. In the book, they said that in such as case, chemotherapy must be restarted three days after the operation, as quickly as possible. But no-one told me this, and then it was too late! I didn't see anyone after the operation, I didn't restart the chemotherapy until a month and a half later. They left me in the wilds after my operation. When they restarted the chemotherapy, it was too late and it had rocketed!

She thinks that the information would have helped her recovery since she could have taken the necessary therapeutic measures.

Patients sometimes feel that their search for information is treated with contempt when the doctor does not deem the information to be immediately useful for the therapy proposed. Mr T, a 60-year-old engineer with prostate cancer said:

> My problem is that I have bone damage. The PSA has risen. It shows the degree of cancer proliferation. My treatment has been modified – they have given me Distilbène. I did some research to find out the dangers because I know that when pregnant women were treated with Distilbene it caused problems for their children. The professor told me there would be no problems. I read the instructions and saw that one should take care with high blood pressure. I had my blood pressure checked and then I called the doctor. I told him I had high blood pressure and he said, 'we will send you to see a cardiologist to see what is going on'. The cardiologist gave me a treatment and told me I could carry on taking Distilbene but nothing improved. The doctor just dropped it; he let the disease develop saying my cancer was not serious. Eventually they did do some complementary tests and they discovered metastases everywhere. In fact, they have a care plan. They treat you at a certain stage, and then, there is no point in bothering and they abandon you.

Mr T thinks that he was not taken seriously and that the doctors treat patients' opinions and concerns with condescension. But he also feels that information is only given if it is thought to be useful for treatment compliance, and that the doctors lose interest in patients when their disease is too advanced.

Patients' desire to hear things in a very explicit manner can become a desire to be enlightened on their very status as cancer patients, in other words to know where they are with their cancer, if they still have it or not. Thus, in contrast to patients who do not want to pronounce the word 'cancer', Mrs R here makes a lot of effort to hear it being said, but also to hear the doctor associate it with the word 'recovery':

The patient: Has it really improved, is there something to be pleased about?

The doctor: Yes, significantly.

The patient: Is there a real reduction in the cancer?

The doctor: I can't guarantee it. Since it could stop regressing, but it could also regress completely, we will see with the scan which we will do after six courses of treatment.

The patient: I thought you would tell me today!

The doctor: No, we have to be pragmatic. We need to see how the images and markers develop. The intermediary scan will show if we need to keep going. The markers have gone down but they are not yet stable.

The patient: Does that mean I still have cancer?

The doctor: I can't say today for sure.

This patient's need to hear the word cancer does not mean she disassociates this term with the idea of 'death' or at least with extreme seriousness (as it is often associated[1]), and this is precisely the reason she wants to know if she is clear of this danger or not.

For some, the desire to be informed is also based on the desire to be able to organise their future, the time they have left and their life. As a result of this, some patients would like to know everything, even the prognosis, even the worst case scenario, in order to be able to 'organise oneself to die'. 'When I knew that my days were numbered, I decided to have a villa built for disabled people in wheelchairs, to do something good before I died. I know the materials well, I know how to make concrete and tarmac!'

---

1 In this regard, the idea of death which is normally associated with the word cancer (although this is now lessening given that, as we have seen, this pathology is increasingly being qualified as a 'chronic illness'), is still very present for a certain number of patients, as the case of this 54-year-old shopkeeper shows, who when asked what he knew about his pathology, replied: 'Not very much, except that people die from it'.

The information that patients gain from consultations should however be unequivocal. Patients resent what they perceive to be an ambiguity in the discourse of doctors, resulting from the coexistence of two concerns – trying not to worry the patient and having to inform them of complementary or exploratory examinations that need to be carried out. Ambiguous information creates anxiety and fear in patients who believe that something is being hidden from them. This is how the patient feels in the following example:

> The doctor: Everything is OK. We have passed the two year point! You know we need to wait for five years to say you are completely recovered. Good, we need to do an ultrasound every six months as well as a lung x-ray.
>
> The patient: Why?
>
> The doctor: Because there could be some pulmonary localisations, we have to see if any cells are affected, it is better to be prudent.

The patient is worried because the prescription of complementary x-rays appears to contradict the announcement of good news: the two year point. Because of this, his anxiety kicks in and at the last moment he asks: 'I have a discal hernia and it is starting to hurt again. Is there a link with my lungs?' This revelation of new symptoms and the resultant questioning are induced by the prescription of unexpected examinations. Patients sometimes ask questions concerning a pain they are experiencing that they would not have asked if the doctor had not announced a prescription for other examinations.

The desire to gain as much information as possible on their condition leads patients to analyse the language used by healthcare providers in order to unearth a clue, a piece of information. 'I dissect everything I am told', said a 48-year-old secretary. The doctors are fairly aware of this and some make a lot of effort to discuss the patient's condition using phrases which are euphemistic, as discussed above, but nevertheless suggest the seriousness of the situation.

Moreover, the information patients are given on their treatment enables them to manage its negative effects. This is not a case of information being used for practical ends in order to ensure better treatment adherence or better compliance but in order to allow them to manage the consequences better, in psychological terms. Mrs N (a 44-year-old secretary with breast cancer) explained how she managed the information that her chemotherapy would make her hair fall out:

> The doctor said that the chemo would make my hair fall out. He told me straight away: 'This chemotherapy is generally well tolerated but you will lose your hair'. He was very definite. And so, my husband shaved my head just before my first treatment. He shaved it

all off. I wanted to pre-empt it. I wanted to decide for myself the moment when I had no hair rather than waiting for it to fall and finding it on my pillow! My daughter helped to shave it, she was playing at being a hairdresser – they left just 4mm. My husband shaved his head too in solidarity. He had quite long hair. I was the one who shaved him. I had my hair shaved again before the second treatment. Normally, it starts to fall out between the first and the second chemotherapy. I only had 4mm left but since I saw it falling bit by bit, I had it shaved again two weeks after the first chemotherapy. That way I was more in control of what was happening to me.

Here is a perfect illustration of a patient actor, adopting a type of behaviour that aims to help her manage the situation. By 'shaving' it, this patient is not only cutting her hair very short to avoid being subject to a large-scale hair loss (as S. Rosman 2003 observed), she is also removing it entirely to keep in control and be responsible for its disappearance.

Although they are often dissatisfied with the information they receive, especially concerning the diagnosis, patients do not nevertheless dare ask their doctors questions. This attitude is not found exclusively in patients from working class backgrounds, even though it is more widespread in such patients. The majority of patients are very aware of the hospital hierarchy and are reluctant to question doctors, especially those carrying the title of 'Professor'. Mrs D, a 56-year-old financial secretary with a tumour of the colon and sizable metastases of the liver said: 'I know that it's a secondary of the liver and it needs really strong chemotherapy because it can't be operated on – the metastases are too big. They are 9cm long. I would really like to know more but I don't ask questions, especially if I see on their white coat that they are Professor or Doctor. The doctors don't say anything, it is only the interns who discuss things a bit, and even then, they need to be pushed. But we can discuss things with them'.

Not daring to ask for information on oneself and one's own illness is also to feel dispossessed of one's body. In fact, many patients behave as if their body no longer belongs to them once they are in the doctor's hands. Equally, some patients feel like strangers in consultations concerning them. One patient (a 32-year-old, with lung and pleura cancer) asked a nurse if her husband can be present at the consultation. Another (58 years old) arrives at the consultation on a stretcher:

The doctor: The hospitalisation report shows a marked improvement in the bone scan images. In his letter, Dr F says he is satisfied with the treatment.

The patient: I have ascites and liquid in the stomach and I am very tired.

The doctor: That is because of your hepatitis C. I can see you have an icterus.

The patient, who was lying down, tried to haul herself up on her elbows to a sitting position to be able to speak to the doctor more comfortably. She asked: 'Do you mind if I sit up?'

A large number of patients prefer to question their GP, although they are aware that he/she may know less. One patient at a day hospital (a 55-year-old computer specialist) wanted more information on antibody treatments, and in reference to the doctor working in this department said: 'If she seems to be available, I'll ask her'. (In fact, patients often try to decipher a doctor's demeanour to find out if they might be available to talk.) He added: 'I know it won't change anything if I ask her, so I try to bother people as little as possible. The nurses don't know things like that. So I make do with my GP. He doesn't know much more but he dares to ask, it is easier between colleagues. I get my GP to ask all the important questions for me'. Another patient said: 'I will ask my GP, even if he will just ask the professor'. The fact that oncologists can sometimes hold the prestigious title 'Professor' puts them apart from the general category of doctors. The patients see them as professors of doctors, to whom the doctors themselves should defer to. One patient, accompanied by her wine-grower husband, complained of receiving no information at all from the hospital doctors on how her medical care would be carried out: 'We are waiting, we don't know what they will do now'. In response to my question as to whether she had asked them, her husband said: 'No! We don't want to bother the professor. I don't want to annoy him with my questions'.

Nor do patients dare intervene in decisions concerning the modalities of their treatment. A senior executive said: 'I think I have to be hospitalised to have the treatment. The ambulatory treatment is better, it provides more freedom, but they didn't offer me that and I don't dare ask for it'. Others are reluctant to portray a negative image of themselves. One shopkeeper said: 'I would rather not ask doctors questions. Asking questions could demonstrate anxiety'. The patient fears the judgement his question may provoke. Others fear giving the impression that they do not respect the doctor if they ask questions. One patient (a secretary), said: 'I would really like them to include me in the analysis of the scan, and explain what it corresponds to in the x-rays. But I didn't ask. If the doctor doesn't offer it, it is because he has his reasons. It would show too much familiarity to ask him that'. As we have seen, it is the very status of questioning with the negative label it carries that causes problems. 'I think that the doctors are happy when we don't complain. So I would rather not ask them', one patient confided, revealing that she has interiorised the social role of a passive patient and the idea that wanting information and asking questions would amount to complaining.

Not 'daring' thus covers different realities. It can be not allowing oneself to cross a social barrier, but it also involves not wanting to waste the doctor's time which everyone knows is precious and always in deficit. 'I never ask the professor questions during consultations. He is always pushed for time and I don't dare ask him', said a 44-year-old secretary. 'I would really like to know … but I don't ask anything. When the doctors see us, their visits are too quick'. 'At home I would write down what I had to ask. I had loads of questions but I didn't ask them, I didn't have time!', said a teacher. 'I would really like to know what the pain that has come back in my lower abdomen is. Is it constipation or the cancer? But I didn't ask, I said it hurt, that's all. The consultation was over too quickly'.

If patients suffer from a lack of information, it is above all the time they pass without this information that torments them. The perception of time in all stages of cancerous disease is closely analysed in Marie Ménoret's work (1999). Time and duration are fundamental elements. They are important factors in the difficulty of enduring a lack of information. 'The worst bit is waiting for the results. Waiting for examination results and operation results is awful. I feel very alone, I could easily crack up. I feel like I am on a train and I can't jump out', one patient explained. 'The longest bit was waiting for the results of the first operation. I had to wait for 18 days!' said a retired patient. 'The worst thing was waiting, I wasn't ill, I just had to wait − for the oncologist, the examinations, the ambulances …', said a teacher. 'The hardest time was between finding out and the beginning of the treatment. I asked myself: why waste three weeks? Why are we waiting?' But time is also a fundamental dimension in the repetitive nature of the need for information. Mrs C (a manager of a retirement home) said: 'I wanted to have the information as we went along. One consultation especially for that doesn't help at all since the questions come to me gradually as things happen'. The progressive and fragmented nature of patients' questions is the basis of Mrs J's idea of a system that could meet her expectations: 'It would be good to be able to ask questions about our illness by email to the hospital, to a department designed for this. A doctor with the files in hand could answer. We would just need to have a code so that the information is sent to the right person. Medical confidentiality would require that …'

In this sense, the presence of an anthropologist is an opportunity for some of the patients to try to obtain information that they had not dared ask the healthcare personnel. One woman with breast cancer, treated in the same department as her husband who had colon cancer, wrote to me:

I remember that the first time the surgeon came, I was too worried about my husband's condition and I forgot to ask him what was worrying me most and now I think it is too late and they can't answer anymore. It concerns the nature of my tumour. When Dr M did the biopsy, he was very surprised by how hard one part of the breast was, saying he had never seen it before. And so he missed what he was aiming for; the device slipped along this hard bit and he didn't manage to pierce it. Then, with great difficulty, he did eventually manage to get to it. But no-one told me what this really hard tumour was, probably because I didn't ask. Do you think I could now find someone (and who?) to tell me?

In some cases, patients are totally rebuffed when they ask for information. Under such circumstances, if they 'dare' ask once, they hardly want to repeat the experience. One patient, a childminder from a working class background, said that when she was giving birth, she complained of terrible pains to her obstetrician-gynaecologist. He replied in annoyance: 'Oh well, you got it in there, now you have to get it out! Pain is an illusion, it doesn't exist!' She was deeply shocked, and heard her husband whisper: 'I'm gonna punch his lights out then he'll see if it's an illusion!' But she didn't dare say anything else. She said: 'My baby had a heart and kidney defect, I asked them to explain what was wrong, but the doctor told me he didn't have time. In fact, later on, a cardiologist explained that babies' hearts finish developing at 18 months and the defect can disappear. And then after that, it got better. But now, I don't bother, I don't ask anything anymore. We are shut out of their world!'

In other cases, patients can fail to ask their doctor about something worrying them simply through self-censorship. This is the case for a 44-year-old woman with Behçet's disease, who suffers from joint and inflammatory pain. She was being treated with Endoxan in order to prevent brain vascularity, but the treatment was causing hormonal imbalance which can provoke a pre-menopause. She was disturbed by the effects of her treatment and would have liked to discuss it with the specialist dealing with her inflammatory disease but she did not 'dare' because it bothered her to discuss this with a doctor who was not a gynaecologist. 'I have gynaecological problems linked to my pre-menopause but I don't discuss them with Dr E. He is not a gynaecologist and that makes me feel uneasy. He is not a woman either. I wouldn't mind if it was a male gynaecologist since it would be his speciality, but he is neither a woman nor a gynaecologist'. Here, it is modesty that prevents her from telling her doctor about the gynaecological symptoms induced by her chemotherapy and questioning him on how to overcome them.

Communication between doctors and patients is very specific. This pertains to the extreme complexity of the relationship itself, which brings together unilateral relations of trust and submission. This latter aspect is illustrated by the case of a patient whose doctor had a partner she had consulted while he was on holiday. 'His partner explains much better', she said, 'he speaks more to me and my child'. Although she really likes him, she decided nevertheless to 'stay with the first one' since she felt guilty 'going to the other one'. This is a particular relationship in which the possibility of leaving for another doctor is considered by some patients to be an infidelity, comparable to an adulterous relationship.

The greater or lesser extent to which patients are able to question doctors or openly challenge them when they believe them to be withholding information is not exclusively linked to their higher cultural standing. It is also linked to a positioning towards medical authority, by virtue of which some patients are more inclined to challenge a doctor and the authority he/she represents. Patients do not all necessarily fit into the behaviour model expected of their sociocultural position. In this respect, asking for information becomes a political act.

Many patients complain about the silence of doctors and describe the difficulties they face in getting them to impart information, not because the doctors *refuse* to give it, but because they are not 'brave enough' to say it and try to offload the responsibility to a colleague ('My GP asked for a scan because he was worried. The radiologist saw something but didn't say anything. He had identified an anomaly in the kidneys. "You need to discuss it with your doctor", he said. He didn't want to tell me what it was. That's not very brave!'), or to another member of the healthcare team ('I had one radiologist who made a nurse give me the scan so he didn't have to tell me the diagnosis!'). Patients thus feel that some doctors shirk their responsibilities by refusing to give the information on the diagnosis themselves.

One patient deplored the fact that Dr Z was totally silent and never said anything during consultations. One day I asked this patient if he agreed to my presence at the next consultation. He answered, 'No problem at all, on the contrary!' and added, not without humour, 'I'd really like Dr Z to be there too!'

Mrs V, a 67-year-old French teacher, said:

> Doctors are a race of mutes! I had an operation on my colon. It took me six days to make my surgeon talk! I told him: 'I want the truth, no-one ever gives me any information!' The doctor ended up saying, 'it's over; we need to start palliative care'. And then, he told me everything. Oh right, fine. I could sort out my affairs, make some donations, share out my money, perfect! But in general, doctors really are a race of mutes. They type on their computers but they don't say anything, and then if we ask, they get annoyed. So now, I shut up, often I don't ask anything at all!

Mrs V once decided to write a note in her care records to the surgeon:

> Could you please inform me of everything, without any hesitation? I have some decisions to refine, even though I have already done most of the important planning. I can take the blow serenely and with a certain distance now. As a teacher, and so I suppose, a bit intellectually deformed, I cannot agree to a treatment or an analysis without knowing what is going on. As a literary person, I don't know everything, but I need to be informed because it helps me to participate fully. Thank you for your understanding

The message did have an effect, or rather, a partial effect. The patient bitterly said: 'And then, he told me things, bluntly, clearly. It was what I wanted, but he never explained anything! When I asked him after the operation, "doctor, what did you do to me?" he replied, "I took out your liver". That was it, nothing else!'

Many patients talk of their attempts to obtain information as a real battle. A trader told me that his GP had discovered through some exploratory examinations, 'a cyst or a tumour in the pancreas'. The doctor had refused to be more precise on the diagnosis. After several attempts to find out more, the patient ended up getting angry: 'Now, tell me what it is: a tumour or a cyst?' The doctor then replied: 'It's a tumour. We need to do a scan'. The patient commented: 'We often have to extract the information with forceps'. Mrs M, a teacher, warned: 'We have to tear the information out of them, now I turn up with a diagram and ask them to show me on it what they are doing'. Fighting is sometimes the only way of gaining information: 'I hold no illusions. If we don't fight to know, the doctors say nothing'. (A 59-year-old petroleum engineer.) 'I ended up getting the details by putting pressure on the intern'. (A 56-year-old semi-skilled worker.)

In their battle to obtain information on the treatments proposed, patients sometimes develop strategies such as asking the doctors the same questions several times over (that is, during different consultations), and in this way, test them to check if they give the same information every time in order to assess the reliability of the information obtained. A 66-year-old craftsman said:

> Dr R doesn't say the same thing every time. Once, he said there were glands affected, and that they had not taken them out because two of them were right next to the aorta and they couldn't operate there. Another time he told us: 'We saw that there were glands affected but there is no risk where they are'. Yet another time he said: 'The operation would have been too long, we could have taken one out to be safe, but it would have been bad for the heart'. Since he can't remember what he told us the previous time, he doesn't always say the same thing! And so I always ask again each time just to see.

Sometimes this battle becomes a veritable assault course for the patients, they go from doctor to doctor within the hospital service, to see if the different sources of information tally. A patient with pancreatic cancer explained: 'I know that the metastases are transmitted via the blood circulation system, the tumour has become vascular and since there is blood passing through the tumour, the metastases go with it. I have questioned everyone – the oncologist, the surgeon, the nurses. I ask everyone to see if they all say the same thing'.

They do not always win this battle however. Mr H, a musician, said: 'I ask lots of questions but they don't want to answer, and so I get angry. The last two times, I felt as if I was talking to a vet not a doctor, I barked and she wrote it down, but I didn't get any answers!' Many patients give up because their attempts to obtain information, including explanations and not just purely factual data, are often in vain. (I will give some examples of doctors being criticised for not listening in Chapter 3.)

Faced with silence from the doctors, some patients try to extract information on their illness by observing them. This observation mirrors how doctors act towards their patients. One patient said: 'Since they don't talk, I watch their gestures'. Reading and interpreting gestures is done when verbal information is lacking. 'I watched the surgeon's hands. I think he was cutting the liver on the screen imagining what he would cut in reality!'

Patients' attempts to keep a close eye on the slightest gesture and make sure they listen to every word to discover information there which might allow them to unveil the reality and seriousness of their affliction result in various interpretations. In this regard, such benign words as the doctor telling patients about the hospital in another town where they could be cared for can be considered as a precious piece of information on the seriousness of their disease. This was the case for a patient from a small provincial town; when she was told she had cancer, her doctor proposed she be treated in a specialised cancer centre in a bigger town, 60 km from her home. She told me: 'They must have sent me here because it is serious!' One patient watched the radiologist to find out his diagnosis, based on the slightest of words. The radiologist was looking at the x-ray and saying: 'hmm, hmm …' The patient said: 'I thought he meant to say, "it's nothing" but in fact he meant, "it's not great". But I only understood that afterwards'.

Patients thus go about reading into multiple facts that assume the value of a sign. This also applies to the length of the prescription, which they understand be an indication of whether their case is serious or not. The slightest fact, such as a change in the rhythm of a consultation can unsettle them. Thus, during a consultation in which the clinical examination lasts a few seconds and the verbal exchange between doctor and patient is also very brief, the doctor says: 'It's better. We are clearly entering into a stage of efficacy, it is worth continuing. You need to continue for six months. We can do six supplementary courses of treatment and increase the dosage, since you tolerate it well'. He then goes on to write out the prescription and the consultation report, taking some time to do this. The patient watches him. During the time the doctor takes to write, the patient's expression becomes more and more worried and he ends up saying: 'Don't go overboard though!' During a subsequent interview, he tells me his case must be pretty serious for the doctor to take so long to write in his file.

One patient explained he 'understood everything' the day the oncologist welcomed him into the consultation room with a friendly hand on his back. Touching and being friendly and reassuring are gestures often interpreted to mean that the situation is serious. The signs that patients try to interpret (doctor's gestures, length of prescription) are sources of information that cannot be medically objectified, although they take on a significance for patients. Ong et al. (1995) make a distinction in the statements given to patients between instrumental statements and affective statements. The former deal with information given, questions asked, advice, transmission of examination results and reasons for treatment. The second include encouragement, reassurance, approval, empathy and chat. Yet, this distinction, which partly tallies with the notions of *cure* and *care*, is made here between the cognitive domain and the emotional domain, two domains which are nevertheless not dissociable for patients since both can be significant and can provide them with information on the seriousness of their condition.

The role of symptoms

Patients manage information largely by managing their symptoms. The role of symptoms should be examined from two angles, firstly by considering what patients learn from them (when it is the symptom that informs patients of their own illness) and secondly by examining what doctors learn from patients about their symptoms, in other words, when patients inform their doctor of their symptoms. While the patients' first piece of information on their illness is often provided by their symptoms, on the contrary, they tend to think that a lack of symptoms means they are not ill. In such conditions, when their examination results are worrying, patients experience even more difficulty in accepting this information because it appears to contradict their own experience of their body. A patient (a business manager) said:

> I don't know, I feel fine. They found it accidentally. I fell off a horse and they took me to A&E, otherwise everything was fine! Apart from a bit of constipation after a few business meals, and occasional overindulgences, I was never ill. I don't feel anything!

A lack of symptoms threatens treatment adherence since the perception that the patient is being made ill by chemotherapy, because no obvious symptoms are being treated, makes it much harder to accept the treatment. In some ways, it is the symptom that makes the illness real in the patient's eyes. One patient (an executive) is reluctant to undergo chemotherapy; he justified it thus: 'No one told me to do these tests! Normally, they wouldn't have seen anything if I hadn't done them!' His words implied that, without the tests, the illness would not have existed.

Although the discussion of the issue of information generally focuses on the information doctors provide to patients, it is also necessary to examine the information patients owe their doctors. Indeed, in this relationship, each party should provide the other with certain pieces of information, even if they do not share the same purpose for doing so. The information given by patients, partly provided by clinical examinations, largely determines the type of care delivered. It also reveals, as we will see, that the practice of dissimulation is not just the prerogative of doctors.

Patients sometimes give fragmented information when presenting their symptoms. In fact, the doctors are not the only ones who fail to deliver all the information they possess. Patients sometimes present themselves in a highly manipulative manner, concealing or reducing the magnitude of their symptoms. The most frequent mechanism consists of patients minimising their symptoms.[2] Patients provide information about themselves in order to try to lead the doctor towards a non-serious diagnosis, or one not linked to cancer:

> The patient: I would like something to help me sleep, because I can't sleep at night at the moment, it really hurts.

> The doctor: I think there has been a small relapse. You need to undergo another course of chemotherapy. It was very effective last time.

> The patient: I called the emergency helpline last night, the doctor told me it was kidney stones.

> [The patient is trying to make the doctor consider an explanation other than a recurrence of cancer.]

> The doctor: No, it's a compression causing this pain. In my opinion, we need to do an ultrasound.

> The patient: The doctor last night told me it was a small inflammation.

> The doctor: No, no, it is linked to a small recurrence of your problem.

> The patient: Yes, but I had a tummy bug recently!

> The doctor: I want to see if the kidney is very dilated, otherwise I need to send you to urology.

> The patient: But I've already done that!

---

2   However there is a distinction between patients trying to minimise their symptoms and doctors minimising the diagnosis. The doctors' minimisation does not in fact necessarily mean that they are hiding the reality, and can be desired by patients: 'My gynaecologist told me that the surgeon was planning a "small intervention". She makes it less daunting but she doesn't hide the truth. And that is good because I would rather know'.

[The patient is trying to say that it is a small personal problem and not linked to the development of his disease.]

The doctor tells the intern present: I want to see the condition of the kidneys so they don't get too tired. We need to do another course of chemotherapy in the day hospital, [and he gives him the instructions].

At the end of the consultation, the patient is still attempting to induce the doctor to make a diagnosis other than a recurrence of cancer, by giving more information likely to incite the doctor to change the diagnosis he most fears:

The patient: 'That anti-inflammatory I had last night from the emergency doctor really helped!'

This time, the doctor does not answer. He speaks to the intern, says goodbye to the patient and leaves. (Epilogue: the ultrasound results showed a dilated kidney. Chemotherapy was booked for the following week.)

Revealing new symptoms to doctors risks leading them to make a diagnosis signifying an aggravation of the affliction. Speaking of the symptom thus makes it exist and risks making the affliction it indicates exist too. The performative character of the patients' statement of their symptoms echoes the performative character of the doctors' statement of the diagnosis or prognosis mentioned above. If mentioning a symptom makes it exist, conversely, not revealing it prevents a bad diagnosis.[3]

Finally, patients may sometimes provide non-therapeutic information in order to dissuade their doctor from prescribing a certain treatment. Patient use diverse types of argument. The information does not necessarily concern the nature of a symptom. Here it is no longer a case of minimising the symptoms in order to reduce the need for treatment and influence the doctor's decision, but to make it understood that the patient's current situation is not compatible with this treatment.

Mr R discovers he needs chemotherapy, after having had radiotherapy. This news displeases him and he tries to dissuade the doctor of its necessity:

The doctor: We clearly need to do chemotherapy so as not to lose the benefits of the radiotherapy.

---

3 Sometimes a symptom is only mentioned right at the end of a consultation. Once the prescription is written out, patients may admit to their doctor about a pain they sometimes have, as if mentioning a symptom which could be problematic could give rise to a prescription or diagnosis feared by the patient.

The patient: You know, I am not that young!

He does not want the chemotherapy and tries to dissuade the doctor.

The doctor asked him: How old are you?

The patient: 77 years old.

The doctor: At that age chemotherapy is feasible, we will adapt the treatment to your age.

Or otherwise, during a consultation, the patients themselves might make their own interpretation of the examination results, in order to curb the conclusion the doctor might make in terms of the diagnosis, when they do not want to hear that the situation is serious:

The doctor to a patient (an executive): I will see you again in September with a new scan, we need to keep an eye on the liver.

The patient: Yes, it seems I have two *little* nodules, but I am doing fine, I have put on weight.

The doctor: Good, well that's fine.

The patient: Apart from these small thingummies on the liver. (The patient is reducing the seriousness of the affliction by giving it a qualification that diminishes its value.)

The doctor: Yes, we need to keep an eye on it.

The patient: All in all though, in your opinion, it's not terrible!

The doctor: It has diminished well, but there are still two small lesions. They are very small. We are not treating them but we need to watch you closely.

The patient: In your opinion, I am cured!

The doctor: No, not entirely.

The patient: Well yes! Just two ovules![4]

---

4 Note the confusion of the term 'nodule' with the term 'ovule', which depathologises the situation.

The doctor: No, nodules.

The patient looks at the scan and asks: 'Where are they, these nodules?' The doctor shows her. She then says, trying to convince the doctor of the insignificance of her affliction: Oh, that's nothing to get worked up about! They are really small!

Patients' discourses concerning their bodies during a consultation do not only refer to the clinical symptoms of their disease, far from it. One of the effects of chemotherapy most frequently mentioned by patients being treated for breast cancer is hair loss. If hair loss is very important, it is not only because it makes the patients feel ugly, but also because it takes on the status of information. It takes the value of a sign that betrays the existence of the disease to the world (Rosman 2004).

On the whole, it is not rare for patients to remain silent or keep some of their symptoms secret, notably in order to reduce the risk of the doctor making a certain diagnosis when informed of them. Borkan et al. (1999), in their examination of the different reasons that patients decide to keep secrets from their doctors, cite the feeling that the information is not relevant, a lack of trust in the doctor, the feeling of power induced by the secret and the feeling of guilt and shame linked to what is being hidden. They conclude that secrets are a barrier to effective communication between doctors and patients. But secrets are not an obstacle to communication. Indeed, they can also be, as are the lies we will discuss later, a means of communication.

Illusion or vanity of information

Although patients can manipulate the way they present their symptoms, when they do mention them on the other hand, they are saddened to see that very often the doctors do not take them into consideration and that consequently the information is delivered in vain. In this regard, the information provided by patients not only includes pain as a symptom of the disease, but also the effects of the treatment. Here again, patients sometimes give their doctors a piece of information aimed at obtaining a modification in a treatment with troublesome side-effects. On this point, they complain that the clinical information they provide is often not taken into account, or is misrepresented by the doctor. During a consultation, an oncologist asked a patient how his chemotherapy sessions have gone. The patient said he had 'untimely diarrhoea *during* the sessions'. At the end of the consultation, the oncologist dictated into his Dictaphone: 'Side-effects like diarrhoea *after* the sessions'. The patient and his wife exchanged a dismayed look, but said nothing. His wife wrote me an email on this subject a few days later complaining that the doctors do not listen. Patients thus condemn how little the information they provide is used, which would, they believe, allow the doctor to make a more accurate diagnosis, or at least prescribe appropriate complementary examinations.

The criticism is not necessarily always aimed at the oncologist. It may concern the GP, whose negligence is seen to result in a delayed diagnosis. Mrs H, a 64-year-old sales representative, told me:

> I spent four years complaining about my stomach. I had my mother at home, she was bedridden, so the doctor came at least once a week to see her. I told him about my stomach pain. Since I was having problems with my mother-in-law and my eldest son, the doctor said that my stomach pains were related to stress! He gave me Prozac and other tranquilisers for four years! He hadn't taken into account how much pain I was in.

The patient condemns the doctor's failure to take her complaints seriously, particularly the information she gave about her symptom, and she believes him to be responsible for the development of her cancer.

> And then, since I kept complaining and since there is history of colon cancer in my family, he just sent me for a colonoscopy, but the x-ray showed nothing. After my mum died, we sold up and did up a house in the country (my husband is a tiler) and we went to live there. I still had stomach pain, and I was very tired. I organised my son's wedding and our housewarming party. I put on 15kg in six months without changing my way of life. In fact it was because my pancreas was malfunctioning. A dietician prescribed a diet that had no effect. Then, I saw another doctor in the village we had moved to. It was a locum. She listened to me, and sent me for an abdominal ultrasound. And then, they saw the tumour – it measured 4 cm! I was outraged with my doctor because he hadn't sent me for the right tests. I really wanted to insult him! I didn't, but I did call him to say they had found a cancer of the pancreas. He answered, 'You must have suffered a lot!' I said, 'No more than when I was telling you it hurt!' He didn't answer. I felt he was scared I would take him to court, but I am not interested in doing that.

The accusation here, and there are many accounts of this ilk, is that GPs delay sending patients for the necessary examinations or to an oncologist, or do not do so at all, because they downplay the information given by patients. Mr G, a 58-year-old physics teacher, described telling his doctor about a pain in the anal area:

> He did a rectal examination but found nothing. But he didn't do a PSA, which could have clarified things! My doctor told me, 'it might be haemorrhoids'. It goes to show we should change doctors regularly! He completely missed it! I got a new pain in the groin area a few years later. My GP did eventually send me for some exploratory tests – but the ultrasound found nothing. He then sent me to an urologist who did a rectal examination, and diagnosed a prostate cancer that was too advanced to be operated

on! The complementary examinations confirmed his diagnosis (the scan, the biopsy, the scintigraphy). My GP hadn't seen anything but the cancer was obvious to the urologist.

Here, the GP is not only criticised for being incompetent or unable to diagnose the problem, but also for not prescribing further examinations or delegating the task to other specialists, because he failed to take the patient's pain and consequently the clinical information he was given into account.

In other cases, patients complain of not being understood by doctors, linked to the fact that the two parties do not assess risk in the same way. One patient refused chemotherapy, to the doctor's dismay, and tried to negotiate her treatment with him:

If I leave now, it doesn't matter, at least I feel better that with the chemo – it makes me ill. I have bought my tombstone, it's there [she shows him photos of a region she loves, where she feels good – the Causse Noir]. I have had my family tree engraved on it. But I don't want to die of a heart attack! In my family, they all had heart attacks! I want to have time to organise everything! And I don't think the chemotherapy is good for my heart. It could cost me my life.

The information she provides on the fact that she cannot bear the chemotherapy and her fear of damaging her heart is intended to persuade the doctor to change the treatment. The patient had evaluated the risks of the therapy and of not following it in a totally different way from the doctor. To have chemotherapy, was, in her eyes, to risk 'paying with her life' because her heart may give up before she had put her affairs in order. It was thus the greater risk. Here we can see a clash of two different rationalities.

Many of the patients' accounts demonstrate the sentiment that information is provided in vain because the doctors do not take it seriously. One woman (an employee), whose daughter had neuro-Behçet's disease, a genetic disease for which the articular and neurological form had been complicated by an inflammation of the blood vessels that had rendered her tetraplegic, said:

My daughter had problems with her memory and poor perception. And then she wouldn't reply to my questions. The GP sent her to hospital for neurological tests, but they said there were no neurological problems, it was a psychiatric issue. They sent her to a psychiatric ward and asked me not to visit! The doctor there declared it was related to family problems and she was stuffed with neuroleptics. And then, one day, she went into a deep coma – I don't know how long she stayed in the coma. She was in hospital for six months, in neurological intensive care. Then they called in another doctor (in internal medicine). Her bone marrow was destroyed, and she had mouth ulcers. She had a scan and they found a dark mass on the brain. They thought she had a tumour on the spinal cord; that is why they sent her to internal medicine. They told me they didn't know what she had. I thought she had Creutzfeldt-Jakob disease and I panicked. Finally the nurse supervisor told me it was Behçet's disease and she was being treated with Endoxan (a chemotherapeutic treatment). But up to that point, she had only been given Prozac, for a very long time, and nothing to treat her. They only found out what she had when they asked the opinion of a doctor from another department, from internal medicine. I didn't dare ask them why they weren't treating her! I didn't want to annoy them and make them angry! We are always scared they will provide worse care if we annoy them! There is something I had never dared tell anyone: she always moved her head from left to right. I asked her once: 'you're tired of all this, aren't you?' She moved her head and her eyes to say 'yes'. The doctors told me her encephalogram was flat and there was nothing left in there. I told them, 'that's impossible!' and they replied, 'there is no point in insisting, Madam'. And so after that, I no longer dared to tell them when I saw her reply to me. Because there was one who told me I was lying when I said she reacted to my words, that it was because I wasn't accepting the situation, and that it was impossible. And then, she had another encephalogram later and it was normal! And finally, she had a MRI scan, and then they realised!

The internist[5] now admits that there certainly were subtle changes in behaviour that the mother had spotted in her daughter, through small signs, and that the doctors doubtless did not listen when she made this known. For example, he explained, she noticed that the young girl answered 'sideways', as her mother said, and that for a long time before her hospitalisation she gave inappropriate answers to questions – a sign of brain anomaly. The information the mother gave the doctors had thus not been taken into account, and the problems she reported were immediately attributed to a relational problem. The internist, who prescribed Endoxan (an immunosuppressant which is used to reduce the immune response this disease produces in excess) recognises that 'the diagnosis was delayed, and we could have avoided the crisis; now she has cerebral lesions'. The girl's mother laments this situation, especially since she knows that it could have been avoided if the information she had tried to give the doctors had been taken into consideration, since what she described, she thinks, could have put them in the right direction in making the diagnosis.

Although many patients paint a fairly dark picture of the quality of the information they receive, others appear satisfied. However, one phenomenon, already mentioned in relation to doctors, can also be seen amongst patients – the illusion of information. One patient (a secretary) claimed with satisfaction: 'They explained it all to me, I asked everything, I know the whole procedure. I know everything about the treatment'. But, when asked about the treatment she was getting, she replied: 'Well, now you are asking too much!' Although it is conceivable that she does not feel the need to know, we should note however

---

5   Practitioner of internal medicine.

that she tries to portray herself as a well-informed patient, and above all, that she insists on being so, an image that nowadays is socially constructed to be valorising, a construction that figures among the contemporary sociological data to be considered in this analysis.

Mr R however has a perfect understanding of the examinations and the results and attributes his knowledge on his case to the questions he asks. He is convinced that the doctors inform whomever wants to know. 'We can find out whatever we want from the doctors, if we ask questions. The doctors provide information in relation to the questions we ask. Today, everyone wants to know the diagnosis. This is why the doctors always reveal it. Patients know everything today', he said, echoing the doctors' belief that 'they only have to ask to find out'. It is worth mentioning however that Mr R is a research chemist. He is especially well informed by the doctors with whom he discusses the technical details of the development of his disease. Notably, he mentioned the toxicity of his treatment for his kidneys and bone marrow, demonstrated by the reduction in his platelets. Incidentally, he objectifies his case in the same way as the doctors, as demonstrated by the fact that he does not refer to himself when discussing his case and speaks in a depersonalised way: 'A break is necessary, because the treatment is too toxic. The side-effects are accumulating. There was a reduction in the platelets, in the white blood cells. This can't be felt but the analysis shows it. It mustn't go too low because that would be dangerous'.

This illusion of information about everything and for everything is especially present in patients who are close (through links with family or friends) to health professionals. A patient, a senior executive chemist, said: 'I don't think they are hiding anything. I know a professor of urology who trained the surgeons who operated on me. I asked him if I could trust them, he answered, "yes, they are my students"'.

Another patient, a senior executive at SNCF (the French national rail network), explained:

> The professor told me there was a problem around the liver, it was worded as a 'discrete enlargement of the liver', 'heterogeneous structure', or something like that. My daughter is a nurse here, she saw the file. The professor told me there was something up with the liver and I needed a course of chemotherapy. They also did a biopsy but they haven't had the results yet. I don't know why, I didn't ask. But if I haven't had the results, it is because they haven't either. My daughter would know since she works here. And I know other people in the medical world – my wife volunteered here.

This patient thinks he is well informed but, in fact, he does not know that much and does not ask the doctors. He thinks that there is nothing the doctors know that he does not know. Here, the illusion is created by professional contacts. He does not think that the doctors would not tell certain things to his daughter or that his daughter would not tell him. 'I am well informed, I ask lots of questions. Everything scientific interests me, I am curious. I ask the nurses: "What is this product you are injecting?"' Nevertheless, when I asked him what they were injecting, he answered: 'I don't know, it should be in my files'. Indeed, my research reveals that, even among those who believe they are well informed, many patients do not know the name of the treatments they receive, nor the reasons for the examinations they are sent for. Mrs J was asked how she was by the oncologist's assistant, she replied: 'OK, I am not in pain. They took a blood test for a hepatic assessment'. 'Why?' asked the assistant. 'I don't know, Dr I requested it'. Sometimes patients do not even know the reason for the interventions they undergo. This problem is partly linked to ignorance of medical jargon and its uses. One patient said in surprise: 'Why are they giving me radiotherapy? Do they think I still have a tumour? But they did a lumpectomy!' The doctor corrected her: 'No, it was a sample lumpectomy, not a therapeutic surgical procedure'.

The desire for information and the frustration they feel about consultations they consider to be too short (we have shown however that lack of time is not the only explanation for the fact that patients do not ask for the information they would like to have), often pushes patients to resort to other sources, a strategy condemned by doctors, as we have seen, since the information they gather is often thought to be detrimental or false. However, Internet searches are not always done in a wild and disordered way. Patients can be very aware of the reliability of certain websites and the lack of credibility of others. 'On the Internet, they cite a 75 per cent rate of recurrence. The intern told me that nothing is true on the Internet, and that I shouldn't read any of it! But I got this information from the ANAES website, a professional website attested by the HON (Health on the Net) code. So I think it is true', said a teacher. Patients often compare the information gathered and their sources, even though, in some cases, they place their trust in a source that can be doubtful, as we will see further on with a couple's conversation about television. Many patients perceive their use of the Internet to be an act of transgression, a 'crime of lese-majesty', as one patient said. In this example, Mrs R, a 65-year-old executive, feels she has broken a taboo:

> One day, I thought my oncologist was going to beat me up. There was an article in the paper about cancer which said that if the colon or the liver was affected, it had to be operated on. I showed it to my oncologist who wanted me to undergo chemotherapy. He was furious because he didn't like the article, he wanted me to continue the chemotherapy. I made the mistake of telling him I didn't agree. It was my mistake, he was like a dog who'd had his bone taken away! I had questioned his competence. Finally, he did in fact make an appointment for me with a surgeon.

The important role played by the Internet in processing medical knowledge and in the relationships people have with information is shown by Hardey (2004), who believes that the Internet does not only produce more thoughtful patients, who do not put all their trust in conventional sources of authority, but that it allows them to question and challenge the opinions of healthcare professionals. However, such an analysis leads to the assumption that consulting the Internet is a challenge to medical authority. Yet this strategy is sometimes in fact the consequence of patients recognising this authority and the hierarchical position that comes with it, which induces them either to not dare ask for information from those who represent such authority, or to ask their doctor to confirm what they have read online.

Following Giddens (1991) who believes that the volume of information available today reflects the diversity of authorities, promotes the emergence of a new knowledge and creates numerous social relations, Hardey notes a reconfiguration in the doctor–patient relationship to the extent that patients are no longer the passive receivers of professional expertise as described by Parsons (1951), but individuals endowed with a certain expertise which makes them partially capable of discussing with their doctor, taking decisions and challenging certain principles in terms of care, thus affirming their autonomy. The observations of Wyatt et al. (2004) appears more realistic however. They write that the figure of an active, autonomous patient who is capable of critically evaluating information and able to discuss the therapeutic decisions offered by doctors, which is emblematic of discourse on the Internet, is very marginal. They remark that the Internet simply amplifies the means of action and thought of those who take a critical, distanced position from dominant medical discourse.

In reality, many patients notice a difference between the information gathered on the Internet, which is general and theoretical, and the information they gather during a consultation, which is specific and concrete. From this point of view, there is no true competition between the two sources of information since they are not of the same nature. However, very few patients would be able to say which type of information is more valuable *to them*, considering the fact that they often suspect the specific information they receive during a consultation to be false and deceptive.[6]

There are cases however where patients are perfectly happy with this dissimulation. The following example shows a patient who is aware of the

---

6 The resulting caution has the consequence that, although patients now have direct access to the medical files, in reality, they rarely ask for them, not only convinced that they would not understand what is written, but also that the information concealed from them would not be written in the file.

doctor's dissimulation. Mrs E is an English teacher suffering from polyarthritis. She said:

> During the first consultation, they told me the pain was in my head, they treated me as if I was mad. It was dreadful, they were making fun of me. Since they didn't find it, they told me it was psychosomatic! I didn't go back to be treated for a long time. It made me very distrustful of the medical body. And then I saw another doctor, who told me it was inflammatory rheumatism. But the treatment he gave me didn't work. He ended up sending me to an internist. There, they found a genetic disease; I have HLA B27.[7] Today the professor is treating me with Methotrexate. It is a very strong anti-inflammatory, which carries the risk of weakening the immune system and increases the risk of cancer in the long term and at high doses. The doctor didn't tell me that but I know it – I found out on the Internet. I know it is not a mild treatment. My GP told me that he didn't agree with the treatment the specialist is giving me: 'I wouldn't allow my mother to undergo such a treatment!' he told me. They give me Methotrexate through an intramuscular injection plus analgesics when my spinal column hurts too much. But I am happy because it has alleviated the pain. I didn't tell the professor that I knew about the risks because I don't want him to think I don't want it and to stop the prescription.

For his part, the internist justified the treatment thus:

> She has intolerable pain, her doctor has underestimated this; he said it was inflammatory rheumatism but in fact it needs a much stronger treatment. She carries a genetic predisposition for this illness, the blood test showed that. There is no point in telling her about the risks to the treatment. She just needs to take it.

On the other hand, some patients consider the information given to them relating to the diagnosis to be useless because they already know what is wrong with them. Here we find the same idea, shared by doctors, of patients 'feeling' what they have, implying there is no need for the doctor to spell it out. Mrs L, a 64-year-old receptionist, said: 'After developing stomach pains and intestinal malfunction, I went for an ultrasound. The doctor said he could see a tumour. He told me because I asked him, but I would have guessed anyway'. Others, who discovered their diagnosis directly after their examinations, which sometimes occurs when the examinations are carried out in the private sector, complain about the lack of support for patients at the time they become aware of their results.

Mrs G, a 58-year-old with no profession, whose husband is an ex-army Major, said: 'I had a mammography and they discovered I had breast cancer.

---

7   An antigene found in a large number of people suffering from ankylosing spondylarthritis, inflammatory rheumatism affecting the vertebral column and peripheral joints.

I found out immediately after the test'. (Her husband interrupts her:) 'It was a radiology centre, people are crammed in there, it's anonymous; they gave us the x-ray without saying anything! We read the result ourselves and we saw it! They had written that there was something causing concern! We understood! We announced it ourselves to the doctor'.

Others again believe that the contents of the therapeutic information given by doctors is of no interest since, they believe, the doctors have no knowledge to transmit. These patients are rarer but deserve attention in the interests of accurately representing the variety of opinions expressed during this research. One computer specialist (62 years old) stated:

> In fact, the doctors don't know much about cancer; they don't know how to cure it. They try out a drug saying, 'let's see if it works'. If not, they pick a different one at random. I thought it would be like an antibiotic therapy. I expected them to do an analysis to find out if the medicine will work, as they do for antibiotics! I used to do a lot of research on the Internet, but not anymore, there is no point! They promise us the moon in 20 years' time. There are different protocols, but they don't know why some work and others don't. They don't know!! The day hospital doctors for a start are not the most competent! When someone gets better, it's a miracle, no-one knows why. I have been cured, but it's a miracle!

This man thinks that if the doctors say nothing to their patients, it is because they have nothing to say. He does not denounce the way they use their power but their lack of knowledge in the first place. On this point, another patient who discovered from a publication on cancer that her doctors had not proposed the appropriate treatment for her case, also doubted the doctor's knowledge: 'The doctors don't know, they are not informed! I suppose they don't read much; they haven't got time!'

Many patients think that information, even statistical data, has no value since it has not stopped them from being ill. Mrs G (a 67-year-old housewife, whose husband is an agricultural engineer) has cancer of the uterus as well as of the breast and lung, she said bitterly: 'They tell us we shouldn't smoke to avoid getting lung cancer! I have never smoked, never drunk alcohol, never partied! I don't believe anything I'm told. In the journals, it's the same. We have nothing medical in the house, no books! What's the use of doing research?' Her distrust and rejection of information are linked to the discrepancy between what she has learnt in theory, and what she has experienced in her body. Mr F, a 46-year-old departmental manager in a chamber of commerce, has liver cancer and a tumour in the colon. 'I had a perfectly healthy way of life. Now, I don't want to hear that I should be careful of this or that, no, there is no point. Disease gets you anyway, whatever your lifestyle, and so now, I wasn't expecting it, even less in my condition!'

This belief that information is useless drives patients to scepticism, even harsh criticism, of the discourse of prevention. This is the case for a patient, suffering from colon cancer, who does not understand why she is a victim of such a disease, when she had scrupulously followed the advice on preventing this type of cancer. 'I don't believe what they tell me anymore. They say we should eat organic food, fruit and vegetables. I've always paid attention to that. I led a very healthy life. I did sport for 20 years. And so why? None of that is true. I don't believe it anymore!'

While the doctors are convinced that patients cannot understand the notion of uncertainty, which justifies their reluctance to answer questions about the prognosis, the patients for their part do not accept — precisely because of this uncertainty — that doctors can claim to be powerless to cure their illness. Patients thus find themselves in a situation where the prognosis collides with their understanding of medical logic. Thus, some refuse to accept a bad prognosis precisely because they have completely assimilated the notion of uncertainty that the medical body tries to instil in them. The idea of uncertainty is so interiorised that some patients refuse the prospect of palliative care because they believe that there is nothing to say that there is not 'something else to try'. Announcing to patients that they will be receiving palliative care is to tell them they have no chance of recovery. Therefore it is a prediction of a fatal outcome. This is demonstrated by certain patients who take offence when no treatment is proposed because the doctors are convinced that there is no point in trying. They think that talking of 'palliative care' becomes a self-fulfilling prophecy, stating that there is no hope for the future, a statement that contradicts what they are always told — that the future of a cancer patient can never be predicted. In accepting the fact that nothing can be predicted, these patients do not understand why the doctors have 'given up'. If there is uncertainty, why not continue to treat and why not try other therapies? they ask, within the framework of a logical discourse built *in response* to the medical discourse. Since, from the patients' point of view, there is a certain paradox in claiming that the future cannot be predicted while behaving as if the future is known. This constitutes a true aporia on a cognitive level.

Finally, patients are more, or as much, worried by the information provided for social reasons than for health reasons. One patient (Mrs B, a 56-year-old accountant in a car breakers), suffering from colon cancer, asked for explanations on the new anti-body treatment proposed by her oncologist. This woman is very scared of losing her hair because of the treatment.

> The doctor: So, we have a tumour sample to send to the laboratory to find out if your tissues contain this target. If they do, we will do this anti-body treatment once a week. If not, we will give you another course of chemo with a different protocol.

The patient: Will I lose my hair with this new treatment?

The doctor: No, since you didn't lose your hair on Campto, there will be no problem with the new chemotherapy, and the anti-body doesn't cause hair loss.

The patient: Can I dye it?

The doctor: Oh no! You'd better not!

His tone of voice shows his annoyance at the patient's concerns which he considers frivolous in the context of the health problems she is facing. The patient starts to cry. The doctor quickly adds: I need your agreement to send the tumour sample. We will need you to sign a consent form.

In fact, this patient is all the more fearful of the possible effects of the treatments and the fact she will become uglier, because her husband is having an adulterous relationship, and she perceives the risk of her body being damaged as the risk of her relationship with her husband deteriorating further. Here, the information she requested is not linked to her health status but to the state of her conjugal relationship. In the information patients require, the health stakes are not necessarily the most important; social and relational issues can also be significant factors.

Finally, a certain discrepancy is noticeable between patient expectations and the practices of doctors in terms of information. This discrepancy is both the result of the heterogeneous reasons behind giving and asking for information or the stakes they represent, and the way in which patients interpret and integrate, on a cognitive level, the information they receive from doctors.

Around the Patient

Here, I will examine the role played by people from outside the medical environment, who gravitate around the patient, be they family, friends, colleagues or other patients he/she happens to meet, notably in the hospital environment. The attitudes of the patient's friends and family may vary greatly, and are sometimes even strongly contrasting in the way they intervene or try to intervene in the information the doctor gives the patient, and in the information the patient gives the doctor. But it is also interesting to examine the role played by other patients, in spite of themselves, in their portrayal of the disease to the patient and in the resources that he/she draws from it.

The doctors' accounts abound with situations where families ask for the diagnosis to be concealed from patients, and the doctors emphasise the pressure they are put under to 'say nothing' (implying that they should not reveal that the patient has cancer). Family and friends sometimes act to prevent information on the diagnosis and a fortiori the prognosis from being revealed:

> One patient is due for a consultation with his oncologist. His daughter, a doctor, telephones the oncologist because she knows her father will be going to the consultation that day. The doctor takes the call in the corridor just before entering the consulting room. The patient's daughter asks him not to tell her father that he has metastases. But the doctor feels obliged to tell him, fearing that otherwise he will not agree to another course of chemotherapy.

> The doctor, on the telephone: If we give him chemotherapy without telling him why, he won't understand! We have a protocol that tests oral chemotherapy compared to venous chemotherapy. The patient's daughter: OK, only tell him the cancer is back, but not that he has metastases.

Here we have an illustration of the situations in which a close family member wishes to hide the truth from the patient, and where the doctor tries to resist the pressure he is put under, wanting, on the contrary, to reveal the truth to ensure a better acceptance of the treatment and consequently greater efficacy. The doctor is put in the difficult and irreconcilable position of wanting both to inform the patient and satisfy the family's demands to hide the truth.[8]

The conditions in which doctors have the right to inform the family are stipulated by law. Joseph-Jeanneney et al. (2002) recalls the terms of the 1995 code: 'Information (to the family) should concern imminent death, but not necessarily the exact cause which remains subject to medical confidentiality'. However, in the law of 2002: 'A fatal prognosis should only be revealed with circumspection, but the family should be informed, except when the patient has previously prohibited this revelation or appointed a third person to receive it'. It is worth noting here the paradox of a code that imposes secrecy in terms of a diagnosis and recommends that a prognosis is revealed to the family if it is fatal, while keeping the patient in ignorance of it.

The act of hiding a patient's condition from him/her, while revealing it to the family, contravenes in one sense the ethics of medical confidentiality; thus two contradictory principles exist. It is as if the family is not an Other from whom the secret is withheld, in other words, as if they are not a third party and as if they enter into a state of fusion with the patient to the point that they are

---

8 The situation is complicated further when the family is divided on the issue of the information to be given to the patient, particularly when the family do not agree on how to manage the announcement of the diagnosis. The doctor is thus caught in the middle of these diverging opinions – between those who want to tell the truth and those who do not.

not defined as a third party (who should not be informed of what intimately concerns the patient). However, it is a partial state of fusion since the family are often given information that has been withheld from the patients themselves, thus placing the former in a position of power over the latter.

The fact that the family can be informed, when the patient is not, is in itself a problematic situation in contemporary societies. It raises the question of how to define the notion of autonomy and its links with the notion of the individual, since autonomy can only be conceived of, at least in theory, in connection with the singular entity that is the human being, in this case the patient.[9] According to Macklin (1999), it is not possible to define a universal ethical code in terms of information sharing, since the notion of autonomy does not hold the same meaning in Asia and in the West. In this regard, he refers to cultural configurations that are concerned with protecting autonomy but are not rooted in the cultural value of individualism, and mentions societies where autonomy is perceived in terms of family determination and not individual self-determination as in the West. In South-East Asia, it is the family that constitutes the autonomous social unit and doctors cannot act against that (Fan 1997). Therefore, the common practice in our societies of informing the family and not the patient relies on logic based on an ambiguous interpretation of the notion of individual autonomy.

But, while it is true that patients are often not informed at the request of their family, my observations reveal that doctors sometimes place too much importance on this fact. Thus, it can happen that doctors delegate this role to the family, and in so doing they hand responsibility for the patient's ignorance to the family – while not being troubled by the contradiction represented by attributing to the family the refusal to tell the patient the truth, and at the same time claiming the patient does not want to know. In terms of the information provided by doctors on the diagnosis or even the prognosis, the family sometimes, to the contrary, play a role of incitement, as demonstrated in the following example.

Mrs C is hospitalised with very advanced hepatic cancer. She has stopped speaking. Her GP thinks her condition is caused by the presence of cerebral metastases. He explains to the patient's son that it is 'the end' for her. Her son wants the hospital oncologist to tell his mother that she will die, so she knows the truth. He asks to see the oncologist.

The son: You have to tell my mother the truth about her condition. She always wanted to be the captain of her destiny. She thinks she is just feeling tired. You have to tell her the truth!

---

9 Concerning the notion of autonomy in medicine, we will refer to the Hoerni's (1991) review of studies carried out on this subject.

The doctor: I will tell her, I'll see her this evening. She may have a generalised cancer, but I can't be sure; we will know from the scan.

(Once he had gone, the oncologist says: 'It's the son who should be seeing a psychologist, he is very stressed. And the mother is fully aware that she has cancer'.) The scan carried out that day reveals a cerebrovascular stroke. 'There are no cerebral metastases on the scan', the radiologist says in reassurance to the patient's son.

The oncologist comments on the incident thus: 'The son wanted me to tell his mother she had cancer in the brain. We have to do radiotherapy on the brain if there are metastases. If there had been any, I would have had to put this device on her; so, in any case, I couldn't have lied to her about that. But I wouldn't have gone much further in telling the truth. I would have told her she had cerebral metastases but not: "you are going to die", even if it was more than likely'.

This episode illustrates that many people conceive of the problem in terms of the dilemma of whether to lie to patients about their diagnosis or announce that they will die. They often do not conceive that there could be a means of stating a genuine diagnosis without spelling out the still uncertain prognosis. The example also shows that some family members would like all the information to be given to patients.

Such contrasts in the attitudes of family members can also be observed during the consultations they attend, where they sometimes overstate, or otherwise understate, the symptoms presented. The following examples illustrate attempts to play down symptoms to influence the doctor's interpretation.

Examinations show that Mr J has a tumour in the colon. His wife is present during the consultation in which he is prescribed chemotherapy.

The doctor: We will give you chemotherapy that will target the colon and the liver. We will see after that if surgical action is necessary. We will carry out an evaluation after three courses of treatment.

The patient: There is another thing, my voice has changed, it's like I've gone hoarse!

The doctor: Really? We need to watch that. You could have swollen glands. You'll need to see an ENT specialist.

The patient's wife: Could it just be tiredness affecting the vocal cords?

In the following example, it is the patient's daughter who tries to understate the symptoms, correcting the information given by the patient during a consultation they attend together:

The doctor: How are you?

The patient: So-so. I still have some discharges from the anus and I get out of breath when I walk. I feel congested.

The patient's daughter: Well, you're just anxious.

The patient: I am losing a bit of blood through the anus!

The patient's daughter: Only a little bit, mum!

The doctor: You are getting better, but you are tired.

The patient's daughter: It does take time!

The doctor: I would like to take a little break, the treatment has tired you out; we will take a month and a half to see if that lessens your fatigue.

The patient: Yes, because I am very tired!

The patient's daughter: She is eating and sleeping well.

The doctor examines the patient.

The patient: My calves hurt, they are swollen.

The patient's daughter: But that is getting better; she wears special tights, I bought them for her at the chemist.

Conversely, family members sometimes intervene to highlight symptoms understated by the patient:

The doctor: How are you?

The patient: All in all, not too bad.

The doctor: Have you had a scan?

The patient: Yes, I am doing pretty well; my liver hurts just a little bit, occasionally.

The patient's wife intervened: You are very tired though!

As we can see, the relative attending the consultation is an actor operating as a counterpoint, which involves correcting – modifying, supporting or contradicting – the information given by the patient. Sometimes, the relative tries to dampen the doctor's eagerness when they judge the prescription of the number of chemotherapy sessions to be too high for example. It can happen that the relative thus tries to intervene in the patient's care, by attempting to reduce the prescription of examinations.

The patients and their families do not always perceive the information they receive in the same way, and sometimes the exegesis of the doctor's words takes up a large part of their daily life together. In the following example, a patient (a public servant) and his wife diverge in their interpretations of the doctor's words, each giving a different meaning to the information they were provided with.

> The patient: I had a rash one morning and the doctor thought it could have been related to a medicine, I thought it was because of the chocolates (it was just after Christmas). And then the doctor was looking for hepatitis, he sent me to a gastroenterologist who did a scan. I told him I wanted to know all the truth. He told me I had a tumour on the pancreas which was compressing the pancreas and causing the rashes. He also told me it was incurable.

> His wife intervenes: We could say he was very harsh!

> The patient: Well, I did ask him to tell the truth!

> His wife: Well, it really got to me!

There follows a somewhat contentious conversation between husband and wife about what the doctor had told the patient.

> The husband eventually admits: The gastroenterologist told me: 'Since you want to know, it is a cancer; I can't promise you it would be operable'. It's true it was pretty harsh! [The modification in his account of the word 'incurable' to the phrase 'inoperable' deserves attention, and shows how patients can over-interpret information, in this case, concerning the possibility of resorting to an operation.]

> I then ask the patient: Did he say 'inoperable' or 'incurable'?

> The husband: Umm, I don't know.

> The wife: He said 'incurable'!

> The husband: Are you sure?

For their part, other patients represent, sometimes completely involuntarily, a source of information for patients, both through what they know about the disease (the theoretical knowledge they have) and through the specific examples they provide as to the possible development of the disease. The role other patients play in terms of information sometimes compensates, in the patients' eyes, for what the doctor refuses to say: 'I learned everything from other patients when I was in hospital. Some of them know through their own experience'. The information here is transmitted through a knowledge gained from experience which replaces the academic knowledge of professionals. Alongside the benefits of the proximity of other patients with whom experiences can be exchanged, patients also give accounts of the harm that this situation can sometimes engender. The role they sometimes play can be very negative. One woman said: 'One day, I complained about the pain to another patient, she said, "oh, that won't last, you'll see", implying I was going to die! That completely destroyed my morale!' Another patient said: 'Once, I felt myself leaving this world, my blood pressure went down to 5. A cardiologist did an electrocardiogram, in fact it was caused by the chemo. The patient in the next bed told me the story of her sister who had dropped dead under the same conditions!!!' It all takes place as if the precautions taken by doctors to say nothing that might alarm patients, are annihilated by the words of other patients. However, patients do not all look to gain information from them, on the contrary, some choose to avoid them. One patient, an engineer, said: 'I don't want to come into contact with other patients; I want to get away from that environment'. We should remember that many patients refuse to attend support groups or patient associations, precisely to avoid having to meet other patients and what they perceive to be a morbid atmosphere.

The people around them act as a mirror for patients, but it is a distorting mirror to the extent that they tend to assess their case in the light of others, thinking they can find information there relevant to their own experiences, as if these others reflect an image of the patients themselves. A comparison made in this manner, to the doctors' despair, jeopardises their attempts to explain that each case is unique and that it is not possible to compare one with another. Yet, patients feel this need to make a connection with others, either to conclude that their condition is less serious, or conversely, that is it more worrying, finding reasons there to feel reassured or alarmed. Another patient explained: 'I was much more worried about the chemo than the operation. After the second operation, they told me, "you will have chemo". Well, I couldn't say no! I got it into my head that I would have six courses of chemo because that was what the people around me often had. So when the doctor told me it was just four, I was jumping with joy'. Comparison can thus be a source of comfort ('One of my wife's cousins had cancer of the lymph nodes, he was on sick leave for five years! Compared to that, I'm fine!' said a patient), even when the comparison is inappropriate: Mr C, an employee, confidently said:

> They took out a polyp from my bladder and they operated on my intestines. They told me there was something abnormal and they needed to do a colonoscopy to see what it was, then they had to cut out a piece of the intestine. After that, they told me I had to have radiation treatment, and that it was serious and needed treatment, but that was it. I understood what it was but I wasn't that worried because my sister-in-law had breast cancer; she had chemotherapy and she is still under observation today, but she's fine. So, I am taking this calmly!

The examples of other people in the patient's life can thus serve either as a model or as a counter model, as some patients try to reassure themselves by comparing their case with others they know, while others want to emphasise the unique nature of their case. But there again, patients and their families do not always draw the same conclusions from the examples offered by people around them. One patient's wife mentioned his mother's breast cancer during a consultation, to say she had recovered, and added 'so you see cancer can be cured!' Her husband replied in annoyance: 'But you can't compare it! That has nothing to do with what I have!'

The examples of others can also contribute to therapeutic decision-making, notably in the decision as to whether to participate in a trial. One patient said: 'I am taking part in a clinical trial. For my chemo, they got me to sign a protocol, and then they gave me radiation together with my chemotherapy, supposedly to prevent a relapse. I don't know what this trial is, I am not a doctor. They told me it had shown some promising progress in preventing a recurrence. My daughter-in-law is a pharmacy technician and she has a client who was treated in this way and it worked really well! So, I didn't hesitate at all. I signed up'. Here, another patient's account was all she needed to make the decision.

All in all, patients' families play a very ambivalent role. They can be a source of information with the patients' support or in spite of them, but their influence on the management of patient information is undisputable.

Patients and Lying

In examining the relationship patients have with lying, we must look at both the reactions induced by doctor's lies and the practice of lying by the patients themselves.

The cost of medical lies

Sometimes a lie only fools the person telling it. The lie told by a healthcare provider who claims not to have received the results yet, for example, implies another truth for patients, who may then suspect that something is being hidden from them. 'When I ask about my markers after a blood test, they tell me, "we don't have the results"! I don't believe that!' one patient declared, wanting to demonstrate that she is not easily fooled. But the feeling of being deceived can be induced by the fact that the patient discovers all of a sudden, after a new examination, or during a meeting with another doctor, that there is, in fact, *something else*. 'When they told me there was something else, I asked myself whether they had not seen it before or whether they had been hiding something from me', one patient said. Or else the lie is uncovered through a discrepancy in the discourses of different healthcare providers:

> I found out that the cancer specialist had been telling fibs. One of my ribs was hurting so they did an x-ray, and then my spinal column was hurting and they did a scintigraphy. The radiologist was devastated when she saw the result and told me to go and see the cancer specialist again. In fact, the disease was getting worse but they hadn't told me anything! The oncologist had said 'it's not serious', but the doctor from occupational health (I contacted a Medical Inspector high up in public welfare) told me that it was and they had all been talking rubbish!

Here, the lie does not concern the diagnosis itself but the assessment of its seriousness. The notions of 'gravity' or 'seriousness' do not however hold the same meaning for everyone, since the existence of a tumour can be considered as serious by a patient, but not necessarily for the doctor who may only perceive it to be serious if there are metastases.

For a certain number of patients, it is so obvious that doctors lie that they do not ask questions, believing that in any case, the doctors will only say 'what they want to'. In contrast to the conviction shared by doctors, as discussed above, that patients do not ask questions 'because they do not want to know', is the patients' conviction that the doctors will lie to them and so it is not worth 'asking them'.

Patients are sometimes very sceptical and ask themselves if the doctors have misread the situation or if they have deliberately lied. Their doubts lie both in the accuracy of the diagnosis and in the truth of the doctor's words: 'They told my husband that all was well, and then suddenly, a doctor told us that he had metastases measuring 6 cm in the liver! Can 6-cm metastases develop in just two months? I thought they had been hiding the facts. In fact, it seems it was because they had misread the last scan. The doctor assured me that the MRI said there were no metastases. They're taking the piss!' During the length of his treatment, the patient was asking himself if they were trying to hide something from him or if the scan and the MRI had just been interpreted differently. 'Even when they tell us they are hiding nothing and that they are telling the truth, we know that we can't believe them! Well, we don't know if we should believe them', said one patient, showing his confusion about the truth of doctors' words, but incapable however of assessing the extent of the potential deception.

Just as some patients do not question doctors, convinced that it would be in vain, they also sometimes suspect they are being lied to when the doctor is not actually lying. This suspicion stems from the fact that patients know they are often spared the worst and that they are not told everything. Mr F said: 'The first course of treatment went well, I had Oxyliplantin. They changed it for the second one, they gave me Sinkafu and Campto – that gave me unbearable pain. They told me it was normal for chemo, but I thought it was because of the symptoms and that the disease was worsening and they didn't want to tell me. I know they are always blowing hot air'.

Admittedly, patients easily make over-interpretations in circumstances where the doctor's hesitation in answering questions can be construed, not as the result of an uncertainty, but as a desire to hide something. We cannot unequivocally determine what makes a piece of information or a statement be considered true or not, but the smallest gesture or word can be interpreted as a sign of dissimulation or lying.

More rarely, however, some patients would have preferred the doctor to lie to them. One case I encountered is that of Mr T who is blind and whose child is born with Down's syndrome. 'The cord was around his neck and the doctor revived him twice when he didn't actually have to. He could have said nothing and let him suffocate; nobody would have known! He could have told me, "he died by suffocation, I couldn't save him", and I would never have known', explained Mr T who bitterly regrets that his doctor let his brain damaged child live. Although he generally denounces doctors' lies because they tend to harm patients, Mr T sees some exceptions: 'We can't always ask doctors not to lie! There are times when it is the best thing to do!' He continued: 'That at least, would have been a lie that benefitted the patient'. He would have liked the doctor to use his (technical) power and his status to allow him to escape from what he experiences as hell, and so act in a way he defines as to his 'benefit' (a variation of the notion of 'the patient's interest').

The recurrent use of lying is not without consequence. Various works have underlined its harmful effects, in particular, the loss of trust. This loss of trust, induced by the certainty that the information has been pared down or hidden, exists in many other cases of disease (see Bastin, Cresson et al. 1993; Cresson 2000). The primary consequence of doctors' lies is thus the mistrust it provokes in patients, the evolution of which can lead them to question 'good news'. Mrs V said: 'I got some good news earlier! But I hope they weren't lying! I got on well with a doctor who agreed to look in my files and he told me the markers had reduced by 1000!'[10]

Among the consequences of lying, we should note the retention of information by the patients themselves. A patient, convinced that her doctors do not respect medical confidentiality since she believes 'they always lie', has decided not to tell her family doctor about anything personal because she fears 'he will go and repeat it all' to her mother. Moreover, both lying and the feeling of lacking information without the suspicion of having been fooled, drive patients to consult other doctors, in the hope of confirming or refuting what the first doctor told them, and thus be able to test the veracity of the latter's discourse. Such an attitude reveals a desire to dispel any doubt, or to increase the chances of unveiling the truth.

Finally, the acts of withholding information and above all, lying, are largely responsible for medical nomadism. An internal medicine practitioner received a patient who has been treated several times in pneumology for repeated infections. She is an executive secretary and has built up a thick file tracing the whole history of her pathological episodes which she describes in detail to the internist. She is worried, despite the many antibiotic treatments she had been prescribed by the different doctors consulted (general practitioners and pneumonologists), that the examinations still show the presence of pneumococcus. The internist told her:

> It's true that it is frightening to see a microbe that resists treatment, but it is not serious. The problem is not the microbe itself but in knowing if your organism can limit its proliferation. Everyone has weeds in their garden and everyone has microbes, if we were to carry out bacteriological examinations on everyone, we would find that 50 per cent of people have a pneumococcus. Your problem is more a bronchial hyperactivity, so we need to give you cortisone to reduce your immunity.

Later, he explained:

> This patient needs a lot of explanations. And her pneunococcus is bordering on neurosis. We have to provide the explanations she asks for because she must leave the consultation satisfied, if not she will go and see someone else. We need to curb her medical vagrancy and stop her going from doctor to doctor. Also, we mustn't give her the impression we are not taking her illness seriously, otherwise she will go and see another doctor. The doctors want to get rid of the problem, they prescribe her antibiotics when that is not what she needs! We must give her genuine information but we can't tell her the truth

---

10   While these words demonstrate her distrust of what the doctors say, they also show her feeling that she needs special privileges to obtain information concerning her: 'getting on well' with a doctor so he will 'agree' to give her the results of her examinations.

either. Telling the truth would involve saying: 'you have a neurosis'. We mustn't tackle the patient's conception head on; it is like judo; we have to avoid conflict in the relationship.

Indeed, another patient, with cancer this time, is convinced the doctors are lying to her because of the 'example of [her] husband who was lied to'. Now, she always consults two or three doctors 'to verify' the first doctor's words. But if the acts of withholding information, and above all, lying, are largely responsible for medical nomadism, we cannot nevertheless consider such a consequence to be necessarily negative. Some may think it is not politically, nor above all economically, correct to not judge medical nomadism as detrimental, but it should be acknowledged that recourse to so-called medical nomadism can be beneficial, sometimes resulting in an improvement in the quality of patient care.

Patients' lies

The mechanism governing patients' lies is however of a quite different nature. Here too, beyond dissimulation, we can speak of lying when patients let their doctors believe the opposite of what they themselves consider to be the truth or reality. However, discussing lying in these circumstances, especially in regards to the presentation of symptoms, involves referring not to a situation in which patients pretend to have symptoms when in fact they do not − equivalent to what the doctors identify as hypochondria, and thus a pathology − but to a situation where, on the contrary, they pretend not to have a symptom when in fact they do.

Patients also practice lying 'by omission'. Just as in the case of the information they may give doctors on the nature and the development of their symptoms, the first stage is dissimulation. It is not just a matter here of understating symptoms, as we saw above, in an attempt to render the affliction less alarming, but of hiding their existence altogether. 'I had two bouts of fever, but I didn't tell the doctor. I don't want to make a fuss', said a teacher. 'For two days I stopped the antibiotics for the spots I had because of the chemo. I don't like taking those sort of things, but I didn't tell him', said a secretary. But what is simply dissimulation − dissimulation of symptoms or dissimulation of a bad treatment adherence − in these two examples, becomes a lie when there is a false statement on reality, when patients claim to have taken their treatment or when they state they have no new symptoms. The following examples illustrate this phenomenon which is observable in patients from various social environments.

A patient who is a senior official, does not want a bad diagnosis to be made on his case. He confided: 'My back is hurting but I didn't tell the doctor, I told him everything was fine'. This patient fears that his back pain is a sign of a deterioration in his condition. He already knows however that it is serious since the oncologist told him of the existence of a malignant tumour in the bladder, and metastases in the lungs and bones. He added (implying that it is a potentially worrying symptom): 'I know that my wife would encourage me to tell them, but I don't want to worry her, I told her that I was fine'. But he does not feel ready to hear about a potential complication of his disease, although his sociocultural level had led his doctor to give him all the information about his condition.

The following example reveals the same concern in a patient to not lead the doctor to make an alarming diagnosis. One woman (a sales representative in a transport company), who was operated for pancreatic cancer said:

After my operation, I was in a lot of pain. I had already been put on morphine before the operation because my cancer was too painful. They gave it to me again after the operation, but they took me off it too soon — just one month after. The professor was on holiday and it was the interns who decided to take me off it so quickly. I was a bit addicted, I was having hallucinations, I saw myself skiing on the TV, but they took me off it too quickly! But since I was still in a lot of pain, I took morphine in secret. When it hurt, I took a pill, one and at any time, when normally you would take two, at regular intervals, one at 8am and one at 8pm. Since it didn't have any effect, I then took two. I was scared of becoming a druggie. I hid it in the bedside table. I cried because I was feeling guilty. I lied to my husband and to the doctor too: I told them it was doing fine. And then I cried too because I was scared that the disease was coming back; if I was suffering so much maybe it was because the operation hadn't worked! When I was crying, I pretended to be asleep if my husband or my children came in. One day, my husband saw that I wasn't asleep and that I was crying. He asked me why, I confessed that I was taking morphine, that I thought the doctor didn't want to give me any, and that was why I was taking it in secret. Then my husband urged me to tell my GP, but I didn't want to confess I was still suffering so much after the operation. I ended up telling him. In fact, it was the normal after-effects of the operation, the doctor explained afterwards. It was normal to feel this pain since my ribs had been opened during the operation. It was the professor who explained that to my GP. But I thought it was because the operation had failed.

This account illustrates the reasons the patient lied and claimed everything was fine, when in fact she was suffering terribly. To admit to pain (she talks of 'confessing' her suffering), is to make the affliction exist and to make what she believed to be the failure of the therapy real. Her lie thus aimed to check this failure. Here, it is the performative character of lying that the patient tried to put to work

In other cases, the doctor–patient relationship is based on a dialectic of dissimulations and lies from both sides. One patient (a cleaner) suffers from rheumatoid polyarthritis caused by lupus (an inflammatory illness linked to an over-active immune system, potentially serious since it can affect the vital organs). In this patient, the disease targets her joints, blood cells and liver. Moreover, she has pain in the right side of the face, which leads the doctor to suspect the lupus is causing an attack on the nervous system. Her doctor is treating her with 15 mg of cortisone. He recommends not reducing the dosage but the patient has reduced her treatment to 12 mg.

During a consultation the doctor is in despair: 'I don't know how to do this because you are not following the treatment as you should, I can't make you better without your help'. In her doctor's absence, she confides:

> It hurts and I got heart problems; the anti-inflammatories are doing some good but the cortisone makes me swell up. I decided to reduce that because I don't like taking it every day. In any case, I don't like medicines. Even the pill, I don't like, I'd rather take nothing at all.

Indeed, she doesn't take the pill but hides the fact from her doctor, fearing, she says, she will be 'shouted at' because this will confirm in the doctor's eyes that she does not like medicines and she does not follow his prescriptions. She adds:

> I do two hours of sport a day, I love that! I do fitness training, abs-gluts and cardio workouts; but I don't want to tell the doctor, I am scared he will stop me doing it! It might not be good for me.

For his part, the doctor says in the patient's absence:

> This patient is not looking for information, she has an inadequate cultural level and she misses appointments. She is quite fanciful in the treatment of her disease. She doesn't follow my advice. She has reduced her treatment herself, which has caused a relapse! In fact, we don't know if it is the effect of the lupus or bad treatment adherence, but it is getting worse. I want to tell her enough so she will follow the treatment but not too much so as not to worry her. I don't know if I should take the risk of scaring her or just be reassuring. I don't understand her. I have decided to put her in hospital and give her less autonomy because she doesn't follow my advice. We need to watch her more closely.

The doctor does not know that she is not taking any contraceptives and believes her disease could be aggravated by a pregnancy. During a consultation, he explained to her, in case she was considering getting pregnant, that it should be planned and that the disease should first be stabilised. In her absence, he clarifies:

> If she got pregnant now, it would be a disaster, she would risk accelerating the disease, her organs could be attacked or she could risk losing the child. We would have to give her massive doses of cortisone.

However, he did not tell her this, 'so as not to worry her'. On one hand, the patient hides her practice of sport which she thinks might be harming her health status, fearing that the doctor might ban her from doing it. On the other hand, she also hides from him that she is not taking any contraception when he believes that she is, especially since he has explained the risks of pregnancy to her.

All these examples show how thin the line between dissimulation and lying is in the attitudes of patients, and that the two practices are found in varied social and cultural environments. However, it is noticeable that the lies of patients and those of doctors are not underpinned by the same mechanisms, and that the modalities and the motivations for lying are linked to the structural dimension of the doctor–patient relationship. There exists a certain asymmetry between them since the doctors generally tell lies to benefit the patients – at least explicitly – while patients lie for their own benefit. However, while doctors lie more often to people with a lower social status, conversely and symmetrically, patients with this status lie more often to doctors. The discrepancy between the social statuses of each actor, or between the social and cultural capital each assumes the other possesses, builds *a priori* the conditions in which lies are accomplished.

Chapter 3
'Misunderstandings'

Therapeutics and Clinical Trials

Among the different stages patients pass through in their medical care, it is during their treatment that the role of information becomes fundamental, in particular when it is experimental and administered within the framework of what are known as clinical trials. The issue addressed in the context of this research, not only considers what types of information are given about these clinical trials, and what types of information are understood, but also what meaning to assign to the situation of choice involved in asking patients for their consent, in the framework of an investigation into whether the consent given is truly informed.

The information to be given on the proposed therapy is strictly governed by legislation which stipulates the need to gain the patient's consent. In the Code of Medical Ethics (1995) for example, consent is the corner stone of the doctor–patient relationship, but this is also included in art. L. 1111-4 of the Code of Public Health, which says: 'No medical act or treatment can be practiced without the free and informed consent of the person and this consent can be retracted at any time'. In order to carry out a trial, the patient's signature must thus be obtained to ensure legal protection for the doctors.[1] Consequently it is the responsibility of the medical body to clearly explain to patients what is involved and furnish them with a written document that provides information concerning these trials, their principles and the patient's rights on the subject.

Doctors are generally very scrupulous in fulfilling this task, which can prove difficult considering how little medical knowledge some patients possess. Actually, not everyone receives identical information, even when dealing with the same doctor. For example, Mr G, a storekeeper, was simply told by his oncologist that he would be trying out a new medicine which is not yet on the market but is very promising, whereas, after his chemotherapeutic treatment, Mr C, an engineer, was proposed a clinical trial involving the use of an anti-

---

1 By obtaining a signed agreement, the doctors are protected against legal proceedings, and in this way are able to demonstrate, if necessary, that the patient was well informed, in accordance with the recommendations of the Hédreul Judgment (25 February 1997), which stipulates: 'In the case of a dispute, it is the doctor and not the patient, who holds the burden of proof to show the latter was informed of the treatment risks or the investigation proposed'.

body that acts on the growth of the tumour. The doctor explained that he planned to carry out an EGF test to test the receptors in order to find out if this anti-body can be used in his case, since it is only usable if the receptor is present in the tumour removed. The oncologist explained the same thing to another patient, a teacher, adding that he was uncomfortable with proposing the new treatment. He said: 'What is bothering me is that this product is used alongside Campto which you tolerate badly, so I don't like giving it to you'. Whereas to a long-term unemployed patient experiencing the same difficulties in tolerating Campto, he simply said: 'We are going to do some tests to see if we can find something that suits you better'.

Indeed, some patients are told that in submitting to a trial of this type, they will evidently also receive another treatment at the same time, while others are not given this detail, which leads them to conceive of the trial as a sort of Russian roulette, a nasty game in which one either gets 'the good' or 'the bad lot' (we will see the effects of this poor understanding of trials later).

When patients are asked to agree to a therapeutic trial, they must sign an 'informed consent form'. It should be noted however that while patients generally read and sign this form, they do not, however, always read the accompanying information leaflet or, when they do read it, they do not always understand it. In the following examples, we can see that patients often do not understand the nature of or the reason for the clinical trials or research protocols and the accompanying legislation.

Poor understanding of the reasons for therapeutic trials and the meaning attributed to a request for consent can produce unexpected results, in that it leads patients to draw conclusions based on the simple request for consent, which takes on the value of information on the illness. One patient, a 58-year-old wine grower with breast cancer, said:

> It was the first time I had ever had a mammography in my life. And they found that I had breast cancer. The doctor said that the diagnosis was worrying but that it could be treated. He made an appointment with the hospital; he called the professor who agreed to see us the same day, in between two other clients. He was very nice, very comforting. 'It can be treated', he told us. First they gave me very strong chemotherapy; I had to agree to it since it was a treatment fit for a horse (I can't remember what it was called, it was a new treatment).

The patient has misunderstood both the law and the principle of clinical trials since she thinks that she needed to give her consent because it was a strong treatment with particularly heavy consequences. She thus takes the request for consent to be an element of information in itself: meaning that her disease is very serious.

Another patient, with colon cancer, whose post-operation chemotherapeutic treatment did not give satisfactory results, was proposed a new therapeutic protocol using anti-bodies. Her doctor explained that, if she was in agreement, 'a tissue sample will be sent to the laboratory to look for the anti-body target'. The consent was thus to authorise sending the tissue to the lab for this research, but not to take a sample of the tissue which had already been done during her operation. The patient told me later that she was surprised they had not asked for her consent to take the sample. 'They keep a piece of the tissue when they operate. I didn't know that! They didn't ask my opinion on that!' she said, questioning the purpose of consent. Indeed, the question arises: what are they consenting to?

Mrs H, a 56-year-old violinist with breast cancer, was participating in a research protocol on the p53 gene, which aimed to test the links between the gene and reaction to a treatment received. To do this, they took a sample. She would like to have the result of the biopsy. She considers that, since she gave her agreement for the research, in return, they should tell her what they found and is surprised that she has not been given the results, not understanding that it is not an 'exchange of services'. She complained to me and asked me to intercede by asking her oncologist for the information she would like to have. When asked, the doctor explained:

> It is a clinical research protocol but the results are unusable at the moment. This is a prospective study and clinicians are not kept informed of the details. When there are a certain number of failures, correlated with a treatment, they make some theoretical conclusions. It needs a cohort of failures and recoveries, regularly up-dated with the information we give them on the treatment of patients. It is done by a Swiss laboratory, within the framework of the European Community. This is fundamental research, looking at the correlation between genes and therapy. They collect biological data but do not return the results. It is all explained on the paperwork provided.

However, Mrs H had read the paperwork. She possesses a certain intellectual capital. Not transmitting results to patients when they undergo certain examinations within the framework of research of this type sometimes leads them to think they are victims of disinformation on their case. Mrs H does not understand that, in this case, it is those responsible for the clinical research that manage the information and not the healthcare providers at the hospital she is being treated in, and so she is convinced they are hiding something from her. Is 'informed consent' therefore not partly an illusion? Are patients truly informed? And what are they informed on?

Some time later, she received the following letter from surgical services:

> Madam,
>
> I am sending you this letter to inform you of a modification in the chemotherapy protocol you participated in. This letter is purely informative and changes nothing in terms of

your previous or current treatments. Before starting your chemotherapy treatment, the doctor performed two breast biopsies:

– One was retained and analysed in the usual fashion.

– The other was sent to Belgium for specific biological analyses.

The sample that went to Belgium (to an organisation for cancer research: EORTC) is intended to contribute to research on the p53 gene in breast cancers. A letter of information and a consent form were provided to you on this subject. EORTC also wants to use this sample to measure other biological factors. Therefore included in this letter is a second informed consent form, with, underlined in pink, an acceptance to use your sample for additional analyses of biological factors other than the p53 gene.

As explained above, your treatment will not be modified and we simply need your authorisation to be able to carry out further biological analyses on your sample. If you have any questions, please contact me on: …

This letter surprised the patient once more: 'They are asking for another signature to use my tumour in other research. Isn't it strange that they ask me to authorise that? OK for a dead body, for the family, but not that!! They can have my tumour, huh! I give it to them!' She added: 'They ask me to authorise its "use" for a second time because it is the law. I did it, obviously; but in return I would have liked to know why!' The patient feels she has been swindled in this unequal exchange.

On the whole, the feeling is widespread that, after having signed an agreement, patients do not know what happens next. 'We agree to let them try out whatever they want when we sign an agreement for a trial!' said a former social worker. On the other hand, other patients think that professionals do not do enough, confusing clinical trials with medical care. These patients are not only very keen to submit to trials, but even think that not enough therapies are tried. The issue here is the very notion of a 'trial', which can be understood as 'trying' to heal the patient.

Mr J is a 63-year-old sculptor with prostate and bone cancer. He is receiving, as his doctor has told him, palliative care. He refutes this term which he believes puts him in the anteroom of death. The doctors told him: 'We can't do any more for you, except relieve the pain'. But Mr J is indignant: 'Other than pain-killers, they could still try other medicines, if only to show us that they are doing everything they can to prolong our lives and perhaps find a miracle, rather than let us die in the ditch! But that is not worth it financially!' He thinks that the doctors do not look hard enough for other possible solutions and other medicines, and just try treatments that are likely to make profits for pharmaceutical laboratories.

He thinks that they do not do everything they should. 'Don't doctors swear to do everything they can to help patients survive?'[2]

Inversely, patients sometimes understand clinical trials to be a change of therapeutic protocol, as we will see further on.

There is abundant evidence to illustrate the degree to which patients do not understand trials. Following his operation, one patient was proposed a therapeutic trial. The doctor explained:

> We took it all out but there are some positive glands. We need to do a preventative chemotherapy to stop the cells becoming cancerous. We can include you in a therapeutic trial. The product is a bit stronger. We know it is effective, but we don't know if it is more difficult to tolerate in the long run and whether there are side effects. This product is well-known, but it is new to use it for preventative therapy. Before, we only used it when there were metastases. The side-effects are neuropathies, with tingling when exposed to the cold. If it is permanent, the product will have to be stopped.

The patient told me later that he did not understand how it is a therapeutic trial since the product is well-known and its trial period is over and anyway they did not make him sign anything. Indeed, they did not ask for his signature because the treatment was 'out of trial', since the trial had already be done. Thus patient consent was not needed. For the patient, the nature of the trial is obscure.

In the patients' eyes, trials are often shrouded in mystery and obscurity, which they do not feel they have a right to unveil. One patient said: 'Since nothing is working, the oncologist is going to put me on a trial. He made me sign the paperwork. "Whatever you want", I told him. I didn't understand what he is going to ask for. I heard talk of samples. It's a German laboratory doing these anti-bodies. I asked some indiscreet questions!' The use of the adjective 'indiscreet' clearly demonstrates that the patient does not feel she has the right to this information, and provides another example of the phenomenon mentioned above of patients feeling dispossessed of their bodies.

In reference to the clinical trial in which she was to participate, a patient said she did not know what they would do with the sample: 'They don't have the power to decide here. It's over there. We don't know who; it's murky; maybe it's al-Qaeda! (She laughs). When I ask the doctors, they tell me: "they decide elsewhere". Who's "they", I don't know. If I bombard them with questions, they will hate me. They love people who don't ask questions. I know they are giving me Irinotecam but questions just annoy them. They don't want to talk'.

---

2 Not every patient is willing to submit to trials however, as demonstrated by this computer specialist's reaction of questionable logic: 'I am not for clinical trials; I'd rather they try the ones that work straight away …'

We should question whether the consent patients give to these trials is truly enlightened. Many of them do not possess the means to give their agreement and prefer to rely on a competent opinion, or on one they presume to be, either relying on their GP, or on the media. One patient, accompanied by his wife, explained: 'They made me sign a consent form to participate in a trial. I signed but then we phoned my GP to ask if we should have done so'.[3] The patient wanted his GP's approval, considering the information he had been provided with to be insufficient.

Indeed, patients often ask for their GP's opinion as to whether it is appropriate, not only to submit to a trial, but also to take the treatment prescribed by a specialist, as demonstrated by the following conversation between a patient and his wife:

The patient's wife: I read a lot about it all, but I always ask my doctor if it is true.

There follows a discussion between husband and wife on the quality of the information received and whether to question it in relation to its source.

The husband: Well, it depends, if they say it on TV, then it must be true! It's not like information in a newspaper, it's not the same! Only about a thousand people read an article in a newspaper whereas millions of people watch TV! They can't just say anything they want to!

The wife: The intern said, 'don't listen to everything they say'.

The husband: Yes, but she was talking about the gossip rags, not what they say on TV!

The wife: The intern said: '*Only* listen to us! We hold meetings to discuss it and we know better than the others'.

The husband: But I still find it hard. When the GP thought my spots might be caused by a medicine, I told him I was taking the same as what I always took, except that it was a generic drug. He told me that generics are not the same. He compared the two leaflets and found a small difference. And so, why do they say they are the same on TV?[4]

The difference in the points of view of the husband and wife is based on their differing judgements as to whether medical authority is preferable or not to media authority, notably from the television.

---

3 Note the use of 'we', showing that it was a joint decision.

4 We should note in this regard the responsibility of some doctors in patients' poor understanding of generic medicines, letting them think, contrary to information messages provided by health insurance companies, that generics are not as efficacious as branded drugs.

Decision-Making Power and 'Resigned Consent'

Sometimes during consultations a dialogue takes place between the oncologist and the patient in which the former attempts to influence the latter's desire to cease or restart a treatment, even though what can be called the 'medical decision' does not generally fall to a single doctor, if only because it tends more and more to be taken within a group of doctors, especially in the domain of oncology. In the era of negotiation, or in what is supposed to be as regards the doctor–patient relationship, health professionals try to obtain the patient's assent, not only because the law requires it, but also to ensure that the care delivered will be of the best possible quality and to guarantee the patient's adherence. However, how is this adherence assessed?

I witnessed numerous dialogues between doctor and patient where the former seemed to be anticipating the latter's reaction, and drawing conclusions about what they wanted that do not appear to me to result from an objective appraisal. When faced with a choice, patients sometimes weigh up the pros and cons, not only simply of the expected therapeutic benefits of the treatments proposed, but also of the non-health based risks and side-effects involved. Here, I will examine some of these dialogues. We will see that patients are often badly equipped to make a decision because of the doctor's ambiguous explanation of the diagnosis, and the difficulties they face in ascertaining how serious their illness is and how necessary a treatment is, especially a chemotherapeutic one. Patients spend considerable energy attempting to gather the details which could allow them to determine this seriousness and this necessity, while the doctors often interpret that as an attempt to refuse chemotherapy, frequently over-interpreting their words.

In the following dialogue, the oncologist of a patient with cancer of the digestive tract compares the results of her blood test with those from previous examinations:

The doctor: It has gone back up, but nothing has moved.

The patient: … ?
(The patient confided later that she had not understood what he meant, but she assumed there was reason to be worried.)

The doctor: Something is happening but best do some more chemo.

The patient: Pfff!

The doctor: The images have not changed but we should err on the safe side.

The patient, resignedly: OK, if we must!

The doctor: It's not compulsory, it could wait until September, but we think (meaning the medical team) it would be better. There is no rush! Logically we should do it; it means that the disease is moving; it would be better to do more chemo.

[The patient does not understand. Faced with the doctor's caution not to alarm her, which leads her to understand that the treatment is not compulsory, she does not know what she should decide to do and how she should interpret the doctor's words.]

The patient: Oh right. I thought it was over, but if it's coming back … [she says to indicate she is ready to agree if need be].

The doctor: No, no, it's not coming back. Why, it is bothering you? You hadn't been thinking of doing more chemo?

The patient: Can it take hold again in the blood?

The doctor: We don't know much about the kinetics.

The patient's daughter intercedes: Is it not possible that it is hidden and you can't see it? Can you see everything there? (The '*it*' expresses the unspeakable.)

The doctor: The assessment of your liver is good.

The patient: I had a tiny little one in the lobe of the right lung. Has it gone? [Note here the use of 'one' to refer to something which is not named at any point during the consultation.]

The doctor: We can't see anything there anymore.

The patient: Yes, but there was a tiny one that wasn't there at the start!

The doctor: It is an encouraging improvement; we can't see the little nodule anymore. We could hold back and do another scan in a month if you like.

[The doctor wants to minimise the patient's anxiety and show her that the situation is not that serious, but he confuses the patient even more; she is in fact ready to accept more chemotherapy – even if it is without enthusiasm – if the need arises.]

The patient: But could it not kick off again quickly? That is what scares me! If you think that a course of chemo would be better …

[The patient tries to lead the doctor to tell her with conviction that another course of chemotherapy is needed because she fears not having the necessary treatment, while the doctor suggests she delay the decision thinking that the patient fears the therapy and the implication of doing more of it.]

The doctor: It would be more sensible, I personally would advise you to.

The patient nods.

The doctor: If you want, we could meet halfway and wait until the end of July.

The patient's daughter: It would be better for you to do more chemo; it would be shame if it came back!

The doctor: Don't worry; a month's delay is not ... The scan won't change in a month. We will just do a blood test to look at the markers. If they are going up, we'll see.

The doctor says goodbye and leaves the consulting room.

He dictates the consultation report: Colon cancer with hepatic and lung metastases. In these conditions, I propose that the patient starts chemo again, but she prefers to defer it.

In fact, at no point had the patient led the doctor to believe she preferred to wait before starting the treatment again. The decision to defer it was taken by the doctor, while the patient would have preferred to act quickly, as she confirmed to me later. Here the protagonists were speaking at cross purposes. The patient would in fact have preferred a firm opinion from the doctor saying she should start the chemotherapy immediately. She did not possess sufficient information to allow her to take a decision. Moreover, the information confused her since she did not understand what was at stake. Thus she complied with the doctor's opinion who, for his part, did not want to 'force her', he told me later. The choice she is left with is a false one since she does not understand its consequences.

In another hospital service, Mrs C, a 48-year-old executive in life-long training, has breast cancer; she was proposed a therapeutic trial. Her oncologist gave her the information leaflet on the trial, told her to think about it and come back for another consultation in a few days' time. During the next consultation, he asked her if she had thought about it. She explained that it was not possible for her to choose between a trial and a conventional treatment because she feared ending up with an ineffective medicine. She had obviously not understood the principle of the trial and thought that the choice was between a medicine with a proven efficacy and a medicine that could have no efficacy at all. As his behaviour demonstrated, the oncologist wanted to leave the decision entirely to his patient and did not intervene to correct her and explain that she would also be treated during the trial. This dialogue exposes the doctor's total misunderstanding of the patient's reasons and expectations:

> The patient: I have thought about it and I won't be doing it; I can't make that decision! You explained that it was a sort of lottery, so I don't want to do it because I have never drawn the winning number. I can't choose that; it's not possible to make that decision! It is a source of extra stress! Because if the result is not good, I'll be telling myself that I didn't make the right choice!

> The doctor: OK, we will do the standard treatment then.

> [The doctor does not press the point. The patient obviously wants him to decide for her.]

> The doctor: You will have a course of treatment every three weeks plus radiotherapy.

Directly after the consultation, the oncologist told me: 'She is wrong since she has only a 20 per cent chance of recovery with this treatment! But I can't add to her worries!' When asked why he did not tell her there was only a 20 per cent chance with the standard treatment, he replied:

> The trial treatment is harder to tolerate. The patient doesn't want it because she likes alternative medicines (she told me she takes a homeopathic remedy for nausea!). The trial dosages are higher, so there is a greater effect. It is more toxic and harder to tolerate. Rather than a three-week gap between courses of treatment, we leave only two weeks; there are stronger doses in a shorter time-frame. It is called a 'heavy dose' trial – every two weeks as opposed to every three. The three-week wait is based on the body's tolerance; we administer a drug to stimulate the bone marrow; in the trial the timescale is shorter. Since it is a higher dosage over the same time period, the side-effects are stronger. But the probability of efficacy is greater. Eighty per cent of women agree to the trial, but 20 per cent don't; she doesn't want to do the trial. So we are not going to try to make her change her mind, eh?

Here is an example of a serious misunderstanding, because the patient thought she was risking not making the right choice ('drawing the losing number') and feared ending up with a less efficacious treatment, when in reality, it would be the same molecule administered at a higher dose. Her worries were thus the result of being badly informed on the nature of this trial. The doctor, exasperated by the patient's enthusiasm for alternative medicine, did not try to convince her. The patient said later that she would have liked the doctor to have clearly told her what would be the best for her, which he refused to do. She thinks that if he had not insisted it was because he was not truly convinced of the value of this trial, while the oncologist for his part deduced that she does not want to undergo a trial. Faced with a decision to make, the patient said 'I can't', but the doctor understood 'I don't want to'.

One of the causes of such misunderstandings is doctors over-interpreting patients' discourses, which are rendered more ambiguous by the difficulties they face in evaluating the need for a treatment and its urgency, and in choosing one option over another. In the following dialogue, transcribed below, this difficulty is evident in the patient's words. He would like some precise information on the need for the treatment in order to negotiate the decision. He questions the urgency of the treatment but the doctor believes him to be questioning its suitability.

The doctor, an intern, enters the consulting room, greets the patient, opens the file the nurse has just handed him, looks at the examination results and says to the patient (without telling him that the results show the presence of metastases):

The intern: It would be better to do a bit more chemo.

The patient does not answer.

The intern continues: Is that a problem?

The patient, ready to resign himself to the medical necessity: Well, I don't have much choice!

The intern: There is always a choice! We need to see if it is something you are happy with.

The patient: It depends if I have to! I just want to know if it is really necessary because the chemo is awful; it's really horrible. Last time, I had frozen hands and mouth too whenever I drank anything.

The intern: The disease is coming back; there is a small localisation on the liver and a mark on the lung. That means we need to act. In the short term, we need to do some chemo to stop it developing. For the moment there is not that much there, but we need to act. We need to start as soon as possible.

The patient: It's a shame, we thought we might get a break; my girlfriend has breast and uterus cancer. We've been struggling with this for two years now! The tumour was badly placed; I probe myself every evening. And let's not even mention sex! I thought it was getting better, this year it was finally OK, and now, it's all starting again. Seriously and honestly do you think this could wait until after the holidays?

115

The intern: I think it is better to do it now. We need to insert a portacath.

The patient: Tell me when.

The intern: As soon as possible. We will give you 5FU; the product can cause diarrhoea but it doesn't always.

The patient: In my case, it probably will!

The intern: We need to monitor your white blood cells that are going down.

The patient: I don't care about that. Will I have reactions to the cold?

The intern: No, that is specific to the treatment you had before; it is one of its risks. It's toxicity at the nerve level, especially the fingers.

The patient: Could we do it in two weeks times? I am going away for a week, I rather do that. [He is trying to negotiate the treatment timetable.]

The intern does not answer.

The patient: When I have sex, I urinate.

The intern: We may have to do surgery but it's not obligatory.

The patient: I'd rather have chemo than surgery!

The intern: I am telling you that because I would rather you heard it said at least once, but nothing is certain.

[The doctor does not want to be reproached for not having informed the patient. 'I'd rather prepare him for that!' he tells me later.]

The patient: Will I be able to live normally?

The intern: Meaning?

The patient: In terms of food?

The intern: No problem there. I am going to see what we can do and I'll call you. The problem is a lack of space. [He leaves and then returns]: It's fine, there will be six sessions every two weeks starting on the 19th July.

The patient: I don't understand, my daughter told me that is was insignificant.

The intern finally says the word: No, it is not insignificant; there is a recurrence of hepatic and pulmonary metastases.

The patient: Oh right, in that case …

The doctor understood from this conversation that the patient did not want to undergo chemotherapy. Yet, while the patient obviously would rather not, it is also clear that he would rather delay the chemotherapy in order to finally have a peaceful holiday. He was, however, ready to accept if necessary, but only if the need was clearly established since, as we have seen, once he was informed of the seriousness of his condition, he was more willing to accept the therapeutic decision.

We should ask whether the current medical discourse on poor compliance in oncology is not partly linked to doctor's over-evaluation of patients' refusals to be treated. Indeed, it is almost a given that patients are always reluctant to undergo chemotherapy. Yet, observing consultations reveals that patients sometimes ask for a treatment (but implicitly) while the doctors assume them to be reluctant to undertake it.

Mr D, from Perpignan, has cancer of the pancreas with metastases on the liver. The oncologist told him in light of the examination results: 'They have disappeared on the last scan. The markers have hardly moved; in any case, this small increase is not significant. If they keep going up a bit more, we will do another scan since we can't see on the ultrasound. If they keep increasing, we will give you more chemo. But there is no urgency. We can take our time'. The patient did not answer, but the use of the terms 'hardly moved', 'small increase' and 'keep going up' worried him. Later he told me that he was surprised that they were not continuing chemotherapy since the markers were increasing. But he did not dare show his surprise to the oncologist, nor question him on the subject.

The way in which patients understand the treatments offered or the therapeutic trials proposed is a crucial element in the issue of their decision-making power. The literature comprises contrasting observations on the percentage of patients who claim to want to participate in decision-making or prefer to let the doctor decide. Although, for some authors, the severity of the disease, age, gender and education have a strong predictive value in terms of wanting information − Degner and Sloan (1992) show that the lower their educational level the more patients prefer to let the doctors decide for them − for others, sociodemographic characteristics and health status only weakly explain the variation among patients.

According to a quantitative investigation into patient preferences in terms of information and decision-making, which dates back to 1988 but is still frequently referred to today, 92 per cent of the patients questioned said they preferred to be given all the information, good or bad, but only 69 per cent wanted to participate in therapeutic decisions (Blanchard et al. 1988). Those who wanted all the information and those who did not could not be distinguished in a definitive manner in terms of sex, diagnosis or prognosis. On the other hand, youth was associated with the desire to participate.[5] By distinguishing between those wanting to be informed and those wanting to participate, the authors concluded that a quarter of patients preferred an authoritarian relationship with their oncologist over a participative one. In contrast to the works that defend patient participation and autonomy, Blanchard et al. (1988) thus call for patients' preferences to be respected and for an appropriate medical response to these preferences. It should be noted that such a position is imbibed with the idea that being passive is simply a choice and obscures the fact that it is partly the result of conditioning, of socialisation. If however it is true that not all patients claim their right to make a decision (an aspect also noted by Degner et al. 1992), it appears in fact that, in light of materials presented above concerning the conditions in which this 'decision-making' is sometimes carried out, those that do claim this right do not really have the means to exercise it.

Therefore, although real changes have been made in the doctor–patient relationship and patients have been encouraged to perceive themselves are consumers with rights, and subsequently as partners with responsibilities, tensions and contradictions persist in this relationship between paternalism and the patient's right to autonomy. Many of the authors who study this relationship tend to believe that it inevitably follows a diachronic evolution as if it is moving progressively from one model to another, continually moving towards more autonomy and information for patients. For example, Hogg (1999) refers to the different models in the doctor–patient relationship which he situates in different periods during the last 30 years: paternalism (where the doctor is the expert and takes the decisions); consumerism (where the doctor provides information and the patient makes the decision according to his preferences in relation to specific products and services); partnership (where the doctor provides information and the decision is taken by the patient and doctor *together*, a model that some authors associate with negotiation[6]); and autonomy (where the doctor provides information and the decision is taken by the patient, the

---

5 There was the same number of women and men in the group *wanting* to participate, but there were more men than women in the group *not wanting* to participate.

6 When it exists, decision-making power is not however always exercised through 'negotiation', contrary to what an idealist variation of the interactionist approach tends to think. In reference to this, Massé and Légaré (2001) think that, in light of the results of a study on the information provided to menopausal women on hormone replacement therapy, it is more a case of persuasion than negotiation to the extent that it is simply a matter of accepting a treatment

former respecting the latter's right not to follow professional advice, a model which recognises the different perspectives of patients and doctors). However, the situation appears to be much more complex since, beyond these theoretical homogenous models, an analysis of real-life situations not only reveals the coexistence of these different models within the same relationship, but also their interpenetration.[7]

Ills and Words

The examples described above provide an introduction for analysing situations that can be qualified as 'misunderstandings'. Either because they demonstrate a linguistic incomprehension that can occur between doctors and patients, or because they show that many of the patients' questions are not answered. At the heart of these misunderstandings reside problems of language, partly linked to a different use of language which depends on the sociocultural levels of the protagonists or to the use of medical jargon by one party that is not familiar to the other (see Bataille 2003; Hoerni 1985; Ruszniewski 1995).[8] Some practitioners are aware of this problem and recommend that visits to hospitalised patients should comprise of several stages: 'After a necessary technical discussion with other doctors at the patient's bedside, we should then turn to the patient and translate the technical discourse into vernacular, popular language; there lies another truth', explained one head of hospital services. Others believe they can resolve the problem by using language that the patients use themselves. This is the case for one doctor (mentioned in Moley-Massol 2004) who is attentive to the way the patients express themselves and endeavours to use the same terms as they do.[9]

The existence of this unavoidable jargon sometimes leads to misunderstandings, either because of the multiple connotations of a term which depend on the positions occupied by the doctor and the patient in face of the illness, or because of the polysemy of some other terms. During a visit to a

---

or not, even if the patients actively question their doctor about the benefits of the treatment, its effects and its therapies.

7   On this subject, see also Fillion (2003).

8   Ruszniewski (1995) in particular denounces the 'obscure and enigmatic character' of information, as illustrated by the use of the phrase, 'infiltration of annexes by local regional contiguity, due to an expansion of the neoplastic process of neighbouring organs with probable profound pelvic adenopathy' to mean 'cancer of the uterus with invasion in the lesser pelvis'.

9   A position that is not without risk since it can sometimes validate a term which is even more worrying or deceptive for the patient, such as for example the use of the notion a 'real medicine' to mean a 'generic medicine' (see Fainzang 2006).

patient hospitalised with a renal abscess, a doctor mentioned problems with her immune system and relayed the history of her various pathologies (scurvy, thrombosis) to his students. He explained to them in front of her that: 'Her general condition has made her depressed'. He meant immunodepressed, in other words, that she did not have normal immune responses. But the patient understood that he believed her to be suffering from depression, and took on a pained and dumbstruck look. She told me later that she asked herself how the doctor dared judge her to be depressed.

This also applies to the ambivalent use of the notion 'trial' mentioned above. Mr T, a 64-year-old business school graduate working as a director in a computer programming company, has cancer of the colon; he said:

> I had slight traces of blood in my stool. I had an appointment for a colonoscopy. My doctor announced to me immediately that I had an enormous tumour in the colon. They put me on chemotherapy and radiotherapy straight away to reduce the size of the tumour before operating. Then, after two months, I had an operation that went very well. After the operation, they gave me another hit of chemo to be sure, then they took the portacath out; everything was going very well. And then during a check-up a year later, they found metastases in the lung. They gave me more chemo and then they found metastases in the liver that were growing. I had five new molecules (I don't know the names) that had no effect. I understood afterwards that it was a trial. The doctor told me, 'we are going to try this'. I hadn't understood that it was a clinical trial. I thought he meant he was going to try this treatment to see if it worked better on me.

The misunderstanding is created here by the polysemy of the term 'try', linked to the object of the trial. It results in the opposite of the situation evoked above, regarding the patient in palliative care who believes that the fact that the doctors were not trying to find an efficacious treatment was equivalent to abandonment, and who asked for 'therapeutic trials'.[10] This situation raises the same question of how much patients are really 'informed' about what is proposed to them.

Of course there also exist terms that are unknown to patients either because they belong to another level of language, or to medical jargon.

> The doctor: You will have a very simple treatment, once a week, a drip for half an hour.

> The patient: Really? That's not very long!

---

10   In a clinical trial, it is a medicine that is being tested, in a case where the protocol changes, it is the efficacy of a treatment for one patient in particular that is being tested.

The doctor: It depends on the products. We will put in a catheter. We will put it there, so as not to damage the veins; it is a very little box.

A little later in the consultation, the patient asks: when will they put the catenary in?

The ignorance of the terms (here a confusion with the system of suspension of railway power supplies) makes one wonder what possible perception the patient can have of what the doctors are proposing to put in his body.

During another consultation, an oncologist dictated a letter to the patient's GP in his presence. At one point, he said: 'The patient is non-algetic'. The patient raised his eyebrows, worried, asking himself what he could possibly be, not understanding the word, but not daring to ask.

Mrs C is 43 years old and is being treated for breast cancer. During a consultation the oncologist studies her files:

The doctor: Let's see the results of the tests … The extension assessment is negative.

(The patient shows signs of anxiety. She has visibly understood the word 'negative' to be worrying.)

The patient: I thought everything was normal!

The doctor: Yes, yes, it is all normal.

She told me later that she was wondering whether they were hiding something. The feeling of being fooled comes from a misunderstanding created by the term used.

Patients feel great satisfaction when they receive precise information on their disease and can then go on to explain their condition to their close circle. The terms they use to do this speak volumes since they clearly demonstrate the perception the patients have of their disease. One patient explained: 'If the tumour is on the tail of the pancreas, then it is a "caudeal" tumour! That means it is not serious. If it is in the middle of the pancreas, it is still not too serious, but if it is on the head of the pancreas, then, you die within three months since that is where insulin is managed. Mine was in the middle but nearer the head'. Note the patient's invention of the term 'caudeal', the result of a contraction of the terms 'caudal' and 'ideal', revealing her comprehension of the information received, that cancer on the tail is the preferable type.

However, beyond the patients' ignorance of medical jargon, another recurring language problem in doctor-patient communication is the use of terms which cause incomprehension because of the fact that the participants are speaking from different places, in other words, of the fact that their position, outlook and experiences regarding the disease are not identical. The diversity of the contents of terms and the contradictory usages by doctor and patient is problematic in that it is a source of worry for the patients even when the doctor tries to reassure them, or conversely, a source of inappropriate joy, when the doctor tries to announce in a euphemistic way that the situation is not improving.

During a consultation, while looking at a scan, the doctor said: 'It is still the same picture. It has not moved at the oesophagus-stomach junction'. This phrase ('it has not moved') is understood in two contradictory ways. Some patients understand it to be 'a good sign', while others see it to be 'a bad sign'. It is a polysemic phrase, which allows one to speak without saying, or to say without revealing. In fact, the doctor and the patient are not operating in the same register. The patient showed signs of worry, and stated that he did not understand why his treatment had had no effect; while the doctor for his part, appeared satisfied and said: 'But yes! I am very happy with the result: it has not moved'.

An almost analogous situation can be observed with other actors and other phrases. To a patient with an oedema on the brain and a tumour in the lung, a doctor said: 'As regards the oedema, nothing has changed'. The patient answered, 'Really?' The doctor continued studying the x-rays and declared: 'No, nothing has changed. Now we need to look at treating the lung'. The patient told me later that he was dismayed to see it 'had not changed', while for his part, the doctor told me he was satisfied with the treatment since the radiotherapy had had an effect on the oedema. Here, the phrase 'nothing has changed' is very ambiguous. If the information provides no further precision, it can mean one thing or its complete opposite, that is to say either an improvement or a deterioration. The doctor understands it to mean 'it has not got worse' and the patient thinks it means 'it has not got better'.

During another consultation, an oncologist examines the x-rays:

The oncologist: There is a slight regression.

The patient's face lights up: There is a progression?

The doctor: No, no, it is regressing.

The patient (in a suddenly worried tone): It is regressing?

The doctor: Yes, the tumour is regressing.

122

Here again, the misunderstanding between 'progression' and 'regression' is the same as that between 'negative' and 'positive'. It is the object to which it is applied in the discourses of the doctor and the patient that lends a different meaning to the terms. While one party applies it to the disease (to cancer or the tumour), the other applies it to the patient's health status.

Sometimes, a term can be so obscure the doctor prefers to use another as a synonym, but which can induce worry and suspicion in patients because of their perception of it. This is the case for the expression 'adjuvant chemotherapy' which many doctors use between themselves to describe the chemotherapeutic treatment aimed at reducing the risks of a recurrence, whereas they tend to use the alternative 'preventative chemotherapy' when talking to the patients, in the sense that it is used to prevent a recurrence after surgery, in a case where there are no metastases. However, this substitution is not without effect, sometimes untoward, in terms of patient information. Some patients reject the notion of 'preventative chemotherapy' since it implies that something is being hidden: 'It is not prevention. If I am here, it is because there is something there'. The notion of adjuvant chemotherapy is thus better accepted. 'That is clearer, and truer: it says we are undergoing a therapy to make us better!' one patient declared.

Another believes that replacing the word 'adjuvant' with 'preventative' deceives patients:

> I looked it up in the dictionary: it is an additional treatment! One should call a spade a spade. It is indeed more chemotherapy. They want to hide all this from us!

> She complains to the intern: Don't do that to me, the preventative chemo thing. They want to lie to me and tell me it is preventative chemo, they want me to believe there is nothing, but I've checked: adjuvant chemo is not the same thing as preventative chemo!

> The atmosphere is getting heated.

> The intern answers: I know what adjuvant chemo is, it is not for you to teach me that.

> Yet, the intern confirms to her that 'a preventative chemo means an adjuvant chemo'.

> The patient says later: Adjuvant means they have added something extra! I knew very well that 'preventative' doesn't mean anything. I knew very well that there was something there!

Another patient too is sceptical:

> After my operation, the doctor told me: 'it's all good, everything has gone! We are going to give you a preventative chemo'. They take us for fools; chemo is done to kill cancerous

cells! They are not going to play around killing healthy cells! It's a matter of common sense! If he wants to give me chemo, it is because there is something there!

For his part, the oncologist explains himself:

> I talk about preventative chemo (rather than adjuvant) and tell them that it is used to 'increase the chances of recovery', since it acts to prevent metastases. It is clearer for the patients.

Thus, the use of the term 'preventative', used by the doctor because he thinks it is more understandable for patients, but also soothing and reassuring, is considered by the latter to be deceitful. The term 'adjuvant', for which the patient above notes the additional dimension, confirms her opinion that the cancer is still there, and that they are lying to her.

Cognitive Discrepancy and Social Posture

The misunderstandings that occur between doctors and patients also pertain to what can be called a *cognitive discrepancy*, to account for the heterogeneity of registers each parties refers to, especially in terms of the prognosis. We have seen that for the doctors, the level in which they place the majority of the information they deliver on the disease and its possible development is statistical: we know that x percentage of patients with similar symptoms have a y probability of their disease getting worse, or inversely, of getting better under the effect of such and such a therapy, which has variable effect on individuals and their pathologies – a variability that contributes to uncertainty. But in contrast to this statistical reality, there is the patient's particular reality, which is what interests him/her the most when trying to find out the medical prognosis.

The conflict born out of this situation resides in the discrepancy between the perspectives of doctor and patient: the doctors find it impossible to go from the general to the particular to establish an individual prognosis and this clashes with the patients' temptation, to the contrary, to slide from the general to the particular, in order to draw out elements they believe to be susceptible of providing information on their case. Yet it is precisely this focus on one particular case that prevents doctors from formulating a prognosis, since they cannot know, *a priori*, and with certainty, how the disease will develop and the effect the therapy will have. Patients thus want unequivocal information, on the *individual* level, while doctors can only provide such information on a *collective* level. Here there is therefore a tension between the individual and the collective or between the particular and the general, which characterises, in cognitive terms, the gap between the respective perspectives of doctors and patients. On a therapeutic level, doctors however have to combine, in a sometimes necessarily hazardous way, this dual dimension since they will have to use statistically proven data on the known efficacy of a therapy and attempt to adapt its protocols to a particular patient, in order to provide personalised care. Making a prognosis is to reconfigure in individual terms facts that are only valid in collective terms. Thus there are two different registers in which reality is perceived.

The discourse of prevention, widely questioned by patients who challenge its relevance because it has not proved true for them,[11] is in fact linked to the statistical dimension of medical statements concerning cancerous pathologies. But instead of using this observation to understand the fact that the statistical cannot be reduced to the particular, it often leads patients to question this statement, and consequently, the statistical discourse itself.

Other misunderstandings are directly related to insufficient medical information, which opens the door to all sorts of suppositions from patients. This is also the case for the factor of age, which some consider to be an aggravating factor, while others consider it to be a favourable one. A surgeon visited his patient who had just undergone a polyp operation. When she asked him what was wrong with her, he announced: 'It is cancerous, but you are young'. The patient described this episode adding: 'I think that it means it is not serious for young people'. In fact, some patients consider age to be an unfavourable factor; others see it as a favourable element both in terms of the diagnosis and the prognosis. It is a sort of empty box into which patients can put what they please, in the absence of more precise information about what the doctor meant, of which the contents vary and are subject to all possible interpretations.

During another consultation, a doctor dictated his consultation report in front of Mrs S, a 59-year-old suffering from colorectal cancer, a brain tumour and a pulmonary recurrence: 'We can see in the images, a progression of the pulmonary nodules; more chemotherapy is indispensable considering the patient's age'. The patient commented on the consultation by saying that the doctor considered her case to be serious because she was old. But, for his part, the doctor explained: 'Yes, she needs to have more chemotherapy. She is young enough for it to be worth trying'. Imprecise statements are a source of misunderstanding between doctors and patients, and of stress for the latter. Indeed, to say to a patient 'considering your age' does not specify old or young. While age has no real bearing on the prognosis, as this oncologist affirmed, it is obvious however that it does affect therapeutic decisions.

11 As shown above, the prevention messages for example stressed the necessity of a balanced diet, rich in fruit and vegetables in preventing colon cancer, but the patients discovered that for them, even though they had a strictly healthy diet, this did not stop them becoming ill.

Inversely, in the following example, the patient thought her youth made her condition more serious. A doctor telephoned a colleague in the therapeutic trial service and told him, in the presence of the patient, 'She is very young'. 'There are reserved criteria for a prognosis, she has swollen glands. I would like to put her on a high dosage intensive protocol'. For her part, the patient told me after the consultation: 'There is a reserved prognosis because I am young, he told his colleague on the phone'. Whereas the doctor gave this information to his colleague to mean he wanted 'to give her the best chances', as he explained to me later.

Misunderstandings can of course derive from incomprehension of the treatment for the simple reason that the patient lacks medical knowledge on oncological therapy. It is certainly not easy for doctors to inform patients considering that some therapeutic choices are very difficult for patients to understand.

The patient: Are you going to tell me today if I have to have a mastectomy?

The doctor: I don't think it is worth it at the moment. For now, we don't know if the treatment will solve the problem on the lungs and the pleura. If there is no response on the lungs and pleura, we won't do a mastectomy. If there are no more metastases, we will.

The patient: That's paradoxical!

The doctor: No it's not paradoxical. There is no point if it doesn't help. If the disease is elsewhere, there is no point in removing the breast – it would not treat the disease. Why mutilate a young 32-year-old woman?

For the doctor, a mastectomy would be a good sign, whereas for the patient, it is obviously an alarming one. The logics of care differ according to the context in which it is envisaged and the actor perceiving it. The simple statement 'we will remove the breast' thus does not contain the same meaning for each party.

Incomprehension of the treatment proposed is not uncommon. Here is an example:

While looking at the examination results on the scan, the oncologist announces to his patient: 'Hmm, it has increased slightly but we have something that might interest you. There is this new anti-body. Have we not already done the test?'

The patient: Yes! We did and you said that it was compatible, it was positive. But you were out of medicine at the time.

The oncologist: No, no, we didn't have authorisation for the medicine at that point. The trials are finished now. But we only do it if the chemo doesn't work. I suggest you do more chemo; if the treatment doesn't work, we will add the anti-body.

After the consultation, the patient said he does not understand why the doctor has decided to redo the same chemotherapy when it has not stopped the tumour growing, and that there appears to be another interesting treatment (the anti-body), but he hadn't asked the doctor this question.

It is also interesting to see how, within the dynamics of the verbal exchange between doctors and patients during a consultation, some questions go unheard, or are misheard. In fact, patients often ask a question or mention a symptom that is worrying them without the doctor answering or even paying attention to it, or sometimes the doctor provides an answer that is on a different wavelength from the question, not understanding the nature of the inquiry. A patient (a retired natural science teacher), to whom the cancer specialist had just announced the continued presence of nodules and the need to restart chemotherapy, asked: 'Dr M told me, after the colonoscopy, that the nerve endings of the intestine don't work?'

The doctor answered: 'There are several possibilities: either a nurse gives you an intravenous drip once a week at home, or you do it in the day hospital. I suggest doing it here, in the day hospital'. In answer to the patient's question about his condition and the diagnosis, the doctor talked about something else: the choice of where to have the treatment. (The patient did not repeat his question, although it bothered him. In fact it is the first thing he discussed with me when I saw him after the event.)

The question can however be implicit (as sometimes can the answer), as the following example shows.

Mrs C: I am out of breath.

The doctor: You need to take a break. We will stop the chemo for a while.

The patient: But the thing is, my breathing is a problem!

The doctor: You will have to do a Doppler to be sure there is not a tiny bit of phlebitis; it's better to be cautious, go and see an angiologist, and we'll meet again in a month and a half.

The patient: Above all, it hurts when I breathe.

The doctor: We are keeping an eye on it, don't worry.

He says good-bye and leaves.

127

The patient noted she had not received any answers about her respiratory problems which were tormenting her the most.

Another patient, a commercial secretary, with pancreatic cancer said: 'I know what chemo is like because my sister had breast cancer. I know it is a product that kills the cancer and the metastases but it exhausts the organism. I asked about the damaging effects and they told me there may be nausea, diarrhoea and fatigue but that's not what I wanted to know! I wanted to know what it kills. I know that it kills the bad cells but I wanted to know it if kills the good ones too! I asked and they never replied'.

Mrs J is told by her oncologist that the treatment is finished.

Mrs J: When can the portacath be taken out?

The oncologist: You can do it in town.

(He does not answer about the date, which is precisely what matters most to her. She waits until she has left the consultation to repeat her question to a nurse.)

Mrs A arrives at a consultation and says to the oncologist:

Mrs A: The gynaecologist found a small cyst on one of my ovaries.

The doctor: The two breasts are in perfect condition. We will do another ultrasound in two months. Do you have any questions?

In fact, she had just asked one, implicitly, by disclosing her concern over the presence of this cyst, but he did not answer. She did not repeat her question, and left the consultation without receiving a response on this subject.

During another consultation, the doctor dictates a letter to the patient's GP:

… the HER2 is not expressed.

The patient bends her ear, asking herself what that means, or in other words, if there is reason to rejoice or be alarmed. When he has finished dictating his letter, she asks him:

The patient: What does HER2 mean?

The doctor: They are not expressed. There is no point in explaining it to you since it does not concern you.[12]

---

12   This is also a perfect illustration of 'practical information' provision, as mentioned above.

Sometimes the patient's words are barely listened to, or even not at all. This is particularly true for questions concerning hair loss by women being treated for breast cancer. In consultation, the doctor asks his patient, Mrs T, how she is tolerating her treatment.

The doctor: Do you feel nauseous?

The patient: Yes, and I am losing my hair. I know that it is minor, but I would like to know when it will stop.

The doctor: A month after the end of the treatment.

The patient: I don't dare touch my hair, it is falling out!

The doctor explains to her the causes of her nausea, while the patient touches her hair, obviously more preoccupied with the subject.

The patient: After the operation, will I still lose it?

The doctor: Weight, yes.

The patient: No I mean … my hair.

The patient focuses on her hair while the doctor tries to draw her attention to other aspects. It is obvious that her hair is her biggest worry, but the doctor does not address her concern. This aspect underlines the discrepancy between the respective preoccupations of doctors and patients, exclusively based on health concerns for the former, sometimes mainly on social ones for the latter. This discrepancy is also a source of misunderstandings.

The failure to listen occurs at very variable levels. It can lead the doctor to badly interpret the patient's request, or attribute to him/her a demand that does not exist. Mrs B, a 42-year-old, arrives at a consultation with her husband, describing an apparently depressive condition.

The patient: I'm losing the plot!

The doctor: You can't cope anymore, psychologically, right?

Her husband answers for her: Well, the journey is tiring! 600 km in one day!

The doctor: I am going to change your treatment, and give you Genzar. You can do it at home, so you won't have to travel afterwards. It's true you live in Cerdagne, that's really far!

The patient: Are there hair problems with this treatment?

The husband: Oh, the hair doesn't matter!

The patient: Yes it does matter!

The doctor: OK, we will see if you tolerate it well.

The oncologist dictates the auscultation report: … The journey is very hard for her, thus the necessity for treatment at home.

We should note that she did not mention problems with the journey. Only her husband brought up the exhaustion caused by travelling. On the other hand, *she* did mention her difficulty in dealing with her alopecia, which appears to be a much larger deciding factor in the emergence of her depressive state, but the doctor paid no attention to it.

Communication difficulties between doctors and patients are sometimes also the result of a collision between the social roles each assumes within the relationship. The doctor–patient relationship is indeed a social relationship (and not only a therapeutic relationship nor even simply an interpersonal one). The suggestions patients make or the questions they ask are thus sometimes very badly received by doctors, who get irritated when they think they are being dispossessed of their exclusive role. Mr J explained the examinations he had undergone during his cancer care programme:

He told me, 'we are going to do a scan. We will give you injections …' I can't remember what, a product. It is a contrast medium. He asked me, 'are you allergic to this product?' 'I don't know', I answered, 'I only know I am allergic to nuts'. 'You should know!' he told me. I asked: 'Can you do a test to find out if I am allergic?' 'Are you allergic or not?' he answered. 'I don't know, I need to be tested'. 'Are you the doctor now?' he asked; he was angry! 'You are requesting tests? I don't want to deal with you anymore! With clients like you, I'll never manage!' he told me. They tell us to take responsibility, but we get shouted at if we do it. In the end, they did the scan anyway without the liquid.

The patient bitterly described the callous way he was sent packing by the doctor to whom he suggested prescribing a test because he was not in a position to answer his question. It should be noted that, although he has a high cultural level (he is a former architect), he has gone bankrupt and is now alone for family reasons. Not only does he speak broken French (he is of German origin), but also he portrays external signs of a very disadvantaged social background, he is badly dressed and makes his living from second-hand goods … This parameter fits with observations made above concerning the social selection of beneficiaries of information.

Finally, a misunderstanding can stem from the doctor's assessment of the patient's request for information, in that doctors are quick to 'pathologise' this request. In the following case, both members of a couple have cancer. Thus they both act as cancerous patients and as members of a patient's close circle (here, their spouses), with each exercising an influence on the care programme and reactions of the other. Mrs L, an executive in a training centre, is being treated for an adenocarcinoma in the breast, while her husband has cancer of the digestive tract. She explained that she was worried for her husband: 'I am doing fine now, I am simply under observation, but my husband had an operation in June, they took out some loops of the intestine; he has a neuroendocrine tumour, and they told me it was a differentiated tumour. What does that mean?' Here, the patient is puzzled by the doctor's use of a term she does not understand, but from which she is nevertheless trying to extract information. It is the use of the term 'differentiated' that worries her. She thinks it might mean that the tumour is 'different' from what patients generally have, and therefore it is more serious. The oncologist then explained to her that it meant that it is developing slowly.

But of primary interest here, is the fact that the doctor interpreted her questioning of this word as a sign of a specific source of stress to be addressed. The patient then deplored that fact that Dr A and Dr L did not both say the same thing, and added: 'I don't know who to believe. What should I tell my 13-year-old son?' The oncologist answered: 'We can't predict too far into the future; we don't have all of the answers, all we can say is it is not getting worse for the moment'. The oncologist then dictated a follow-up prescription – an ultrasound and a pulmonary x-ray to be done in six months' time. He asked her: 'Do you want an anxiolytic? You could take Lysanxia, until you see a professional'. Then he dictated the consultation report: '… She is very affected on a psychological level by her husband's condition. I advised her to see a specialist'.

It is striking to note here that Mrs L's worry, legitimately engendered by obscure and contradictory information, is managed as a pathology and she is prescribed psychotropic drugs. The oncologist *medicalises* her need for information and clarification. Here my point is not to question the doctor's diagnosis, but to emphasise the status assigned to her need to understand, and to highlight one form of social treatment of a request for information.

All these observations reveal the existence of numerous misunderstandings between doctors and patients, of which language problems are only one dimension. They also reveal how patients' questions and associated worries are often '*misheard*', that they receive empty or inappropriate answers, and moreover, the pernicious role that this vacuity plays in the patients' feeling of being fooled.

Conclusion

On reading publications on 'health democracy' (*Revue française des Affaires sociales*, 2000), it appears taken for granted that, nowadays, the contemporary patient is an individual who holds real decision-making power which is based on ever-increasing information. However, it may be the case, as this study suggests, that this obviousness should be re-examined. The material gathered and the analyses proposed here invite us to question the reality of this information. In the medical body, just as among patients, we can see more professions of faith on the need for information than actual behaviour demonstrating willingness to give it or ask for it. As we have seen, although on one hand the legislation aims to guarantee the provision of information and, on the other hand a certain number of health professionals defend the practice, patient information is still very fragmented, even deficient. The problem does not simply lie in the implementation of the law:[1] the obstacles are not only legal difficulties or delay; they are primarily social and cultural. The difficulty also partly pertains to the social valency of the role each participant attributes to themselves and to the other within the doctor–patient relationship. The changes that can be observed in the last ten years in doctor–patient communication have not eliminated the unequal relationship that exists between them, in virtue of which each occupies a distinct social role. Thus, if there exists a certain tension today in patients' relationships with the medical body, illustrated by an associative mobilisation among certain patients – with social visibility as a consequence – there also exists, as this study has shown, quiet resistance which is mainly expressed through dissimulation. As a social relationship, the therapeutic relationship inevitably consists of collaboration and complicity, but also of conflict, fear and competition. Inside this relationship, each manages their own words and wonders about the words of the other, and each actor tries to acquire power through their use of them. Therefore, lying is an integral part of the therapeutic relationship as it is in every social relationship; however, it follows its own specific mechanisms and modalities.

How the actors justify what they say and do not say has been reviewed and analysed in this work; the analysis shows that information provision and lying take the value of a strategy for the actors. The question of information receives

---

1   For some authors (for example Lahoutte 2000), the difficulty lies in implementing the legislation in civil society.

very variable modalities of response, depending on whether it is addressed from a therapeutic angle or an ethical angle. In some cases, the information provided has a practical, therapeutic aim — to induce the patient to agree to the treatment; in other cases, it aims to answer to ethical principles, and the two do not necessarily overlap; in other cases again, it tries to respond *a minima* to a patient's request, or what is perceived as such, while combining the answer with a lie that can have either beneficial or harmful effects. But the retention of information – or its dissimulation – is also subject to the same motives. So that two opposing practices, lying or telling the truth, are justified by their protagonists in the name of the same principles: the ethical one and the practical one.

The search for information is now more than ever a fundamental stake in the doctor–patient relationship. It mobilises various techniques for obtaining information from – or refusing it to – the other, and structures a large part of the exchanges that take place between them. The roles are not symmetrical, if only because doctors are presumed to lie for the benefit of the other, while patients lie for their own benefit. The asymmetry of their respective roles and modes of communication they use, we have seen, is due to several factors, among which we find: cognitive discrepancy (in virtue of which doctors and patients reason on different scales of thought), the heterogeneity of stakes (health related or social) that motivate their choices, and errors in interpretation of the other's discourse and the resultant misunderstandings. In this regard, the nature of the information received, but above all the information understood, leads us to speak of resigned, rather than informed, consent.

The practice of lying is omnipresent in the doctor–patient relationship. In this respect, we could consider the lie to be an ingredient of the therapeutic relationship, which is designed to ensure its favourable development, at least from the point of view of the protagonist telling it. To extend this metaphor, we could consider the justifications given: humanity, practicality, facility, weakness and so on, as the *indications* of the lie, its doctrine and the modalities of its accomplishment, as its *dosage*, and the patient's resultant mistrust, lack of understanding of the seriousness of one's condition, and medical nomadism, as its *side-effects*. We have seen that lying is a practice which is continually being constructed, both in reaction to the attitudes of the other, the one being fooled, and according to how the situation itself develops, such as the development of the pathology. Thus lying can be practiced in stages, following a complex dynamic that takes into account the effects it produces on the person it is aimed at.

The issue of information and lying is partly related to the notion of seriousness, which is the principal element at stake. If this problem is generally addressed within the context of cancer, it is precisely because cancer is emblematic of a serious disease. But seriousness also concerns other diseases; this is why dissimulation and lying can also be observed in other contexts.

In terms of the specific domain of oncology, we have seen that the silence in the past on the existence of cancer has today been replaced and it is now practiced on the existence of metastases, because of the relative trivialisation of the former, and the connotation of seriousness of the latter. It is indeed in relation to this latter that lies are mainly told today, even though members of the medical professions are firmly convinced that nowadays, the patient is told everything. While the presence of cancer may no longer be hidden, another reality is now often dissimulated when the diagnosis itself carries the prognosis. The taboo has in this way changed object − it has slid from a refusal to disclose the disease to a refusal to disclose its aggravation.

Of course, not all doctors lie, nor do they do so in the same way or for the same reasons. However, lying is, in some ways, a norm within medical practice, although individual practices are the result of actors re-evaluating and reinterpreting these norms. The good faith of these actors cannot be questioned. It is evident that some doctors strive to promote better information – although they are often only vaguely aware of the reasons for their behaviour and the effects it has – and demonstrate their willingness to adapt their actions according to patients' psychological dispositions. However, this research has enabled me to unearth a certain number of mechanisms that function outside the psychological explanations often used to account for communication difficulties between doctors and patients and to characterise their behaviour regarding information. We have seen that in fact this information is as much, if not more, subject to social criteria as to psychological motives.

Beyond the communication difficulties between doctor and patient that result from adhesions to different linguistic codes, it is noticeable that the practices of providing information and lying follow a mechanism of social reproduction, in which the doctors, wanting to adapt to the supposed aptitude of patients to receive the information, only provide it to those in society who would normally possess it or who are more capable of obtaining it. Just as doctors select the patients they provide information to − thus contributing to the existing social inequality in access to information − they also select those they lie to. As Koyré (1996) remarks in his philosophical reflections on lying, lies are expressed by words and all words are addressed to somebody: 'We do not lie "to the air around us". We lie … to somebody'. Yet, it is remarkable that doctors are more likely to lie to patients from a working class background and that the patients from the same background are more often observed to lie. The inequalities in access to medical information do not only result from a lack of competence in the tools given by society to certain patients to understand it, but also from a retention, *a priori*, of information from patients from these social backgrounds. In the final analysis, what the doctors choose to say or not say to their patients is thus largely motivated, not so much by − or in any case not exclusively by − the particular psychology of the person receiving the information and his/

her capability to understand it, but according to – even sometimes prior to considering the pathological condition of the patient – his/her real or supposed sociocultural status. In this regard, we have seen that doctors' attitudes vary, although they may not necessarily be aware of it, not always in accordance with who the patient *is* but with who they *think he/she is*.

Although there are numerous reasons for doctors to lie, just as there are for patients, both parties act, on one hand, from a desire to make the illness not exist (see the performative character of lying), and, on the other hand, from an adhesion to their assigned place in the doctor–patient relationship. Thus, the lies told by each party act as a reaffirmation of their professional and social status. On both sides, the practice of lying allows the mechanisms of power (and of resistance to power) to be played out without taking an overt form since subjects face great difficulty in circumventing the values these mechanisms rest on: the authority of the doctor and the new role of patients as it is constructed today.

The doctors often find themselves torn between conforming to their social role which authorises them not to say everything, and even to lie, and not appearing to be contravening the new values dictated by health democracy that advocate patient autonomy. The difficulty in which they find themselves stems from the existence of contradictory requirements which create the context for 'ethical dissonance'.

For the patients, lying is the result of an alchemy between their adhesion to the model of the doctor as a professional *and* social authority and their growing tendency, if not to question the legitimacy of the doctor's words, but at least to secretly resist them. By lying, the doctors perpetuate the patients' status as subordinates, while the latter partly submit to the status assigned to them. At this level, lying operates symmetrical actions, both as an instrument for reproducing social relations between doctors and patients, and as a means of subverting the new roles that society has assigned to them.

Bibliography

Abiven, M., 1996. Mentir pour bien faire ? Ou le mensonge en médecine. *Etudes psychothérapiques*, 13, pp. 39–50.

Aiach, P. and Fassin, D. eds., 1994. *Les métiers de la santé. Enjeux de pouvoir et quête de légitimité*. Paris: Anthropos.

Aïach, P., Fassin, D. and Saliba, J., 1994. Crise, pouvoir et légitimité. In: P. Aiach and D. Fassin, eds. *Les métiers de la santé, enjeux de pouvoir et quête de légitimité*. Paris: Anthropos-Economica, pp. 9–42.

Akrich, M. and Méadel, C., 2004. Problématiser la question des usages. *Sciences sociales et santé*, 22(1), pp. 5–20.

Amar, L. and Minvielle, E., 2000. L'action publique en faveur de l'usager: de la dynamique institutionnelle aux pratiques quotidiennes de travail. Le cas de l'obligation d'informer le malade. *Sociologie du travail*, 1(42), pp. 69–89.

Amiel, P., 2002. Enquête sur les pratiques d'information et de recueil du consentement dans la recherche médicale: consentir, mais à quoi? *Revue française des Affaires sociales*, 3, pp. 219–34.

Arendt, H., 1972. *Du mensonge à la violence, Essais de politique contemporaine*. Translated from English by G. Durand. Paris: Calmann-Lévy.

Ariès, P., 1982. *Essai sur l'histoire de la mort en Occident*. Paris: Le Seuil.

Armstrong, D., 1987. Silence and truth in death and dying, *Social Science and Medicine*, 24, pp. 651–7.

Augé, M. ed., 1974. *La construction du monde. Religions, représentations, idéologies*. Paris: Maspéro.

Baider, L., Ever-Hadani, P. and De-Nour, K., 1995. The impact of culture on perceptions of patient-physician satisfaction. *Israeli Journal of Medical Science*, 31, pp. 179–85.

Barbot, J., 2002. *Les malades en mouvements. La médecine et la science à l'épreuve du sida*. Paris: Balland.

Barnes, J., 1994. *A pack of lies: Towards a sociology of lying*. Cambridge: Cambridge University Press.

Bastin, N., Cresson, G. and Tyberghein J., 1993. *Approche sociologique de la demande en réparation du préjudice thérapeutique. Le cas du sida*. Rapport. Paris: ANRS/ INSERM.

Baszanger, I., 1986. Les maladies chroniques et leur ordre négocié. *Revue française de sociologie*, 27, pp. 3–27.

Bataille, P., 2003. *Un cancer et la vie. Les malades face à la maladie*. Paris: Balland.

Beisecker, A.E. and Beisecker, T.D., 1990. Patient information-seeking behaviors when communicating with doctors. *Medical Care*, 28(1), pp. 19–28.

Bensaïd, N., 1981. *La lumière médicale*. Paris: Le Seuil.

Bensaïd, N., 1983. Dire la mort. *Le Genre humain*, 7–8, pp. 103–15.

Blanchard, C., Labrecque, M., Ruckdeschel J. and Blanchard E., 1988. Information and decision-making preferences of hospitalized adult cancer patients. *Social Science & Medicine*, 27(11), pp. 1139–45.

Boituzat, F., 1993. *Un droit de mentir? Constant ou Kant*. Paris: PUF.

Bok, S., 1979. *Lying: Moral choice in public and private life*. New York: Vintage Books.

Bok, S., 1984. *Secrets. On the ethics of concealment and revelation*. Oxford/Melbourne: Oxford University Press.

Bolly, A., Dal S., Delavallée M. and Francart J., 1997. Faut-il dire la vérité aux malades incurables? [htm] Faculté Notre Dame de la Paix de Namur: Séminaire de bioéthique Qualité de vie et vie finissante. workshop paper. Available at: http://barkokhba.chez.com/verite.htm [accessed 28 August 2014].

Borkan, J., Reis, S., Steinmetz, D. and Medalie, J.H. eds., 1999. *Patients and doctors. Life changing stories from primary care*. London/Madison: University of Wisconsin Press.

Bouchayer, F., 2002. La construction du rôle de soignant : proposition pour une approche socio-anthropologique de la bienveillance et de l'indifférence. *Santé publique et sciences sociales*, 8–9, pp. 53–68.

Broca, C., 2003. La communauté des malades du sida comme fiction: les associations à l'épreuve du singulier. *Sciences Sociales et Santé*, 21(3), pp. 71–83.

Brocas, A.M. and Le Coz, G., 2000. La démocratie sanitaire. *Revue française des Affaires sociales*, 2, pp. 9–14.

Brock, D.W. and Wartman, S.A., 1990. When competent patients make irrational choices. *New England Journal of Medicine*, 322, pp. 1595–9.

Broclain, D., 2000. Responsabilité. *Revue française des affaires sociales*, 2, pp. 44–6.

Broclain, D., 2001. La place de la personne hospitalisée dans la décision en cardiologie, Paris, rapport pour la Fondation de l'avenir.

Callon, M., Lascoumes, P. and Barthe, Y., 2001. *Agir dans un monde incertain. Essai sur la démocratie technique*. Paris: Le Seuil.

Caniard, E., 2001. Droits des malades, *Actualité et dossier en Santé publique*, ADSP n°36, 20–23.

Carricaburu, D. and Pierret, J., 1995. From biographical disruption to biographical reinforcement: the case of HIV-positive men. *Sociology of Health & Illness*, 17(1), pp. 65–88.

Cassileth, B. ed., 1979. *The cancer patient. Social and medical aspects of care*. Philadelphia: Lea & Febiger.

Charavel, M., 2004. Participation au choix thérapeutique en oncologie. *Revue francophone de psycho-oncologie*, 4, pp. 201–5.

Charles, C., Gafni, A. and Whelan, T., 1999. Decision-making in the physician-patient encounter: revisiting the shared treatment decision-making model. *Social science & medicine*, 49, pp. 651–61.

Collectif, 1966. Le mensonge en médecine. 10ème colloque du groupe 'Médecine de France'. *Panorama de la pensée médicale, littéraire et artistique française*, 177, pp. 3–16.

Collier, J. and Iheanacho, I., 2002. The pharmaceutical industry as an informant. *The Lancet*, 360(9343), pp. 1405–9.

Constant, B., 2003. Tout le monde n'a pas droit à la vérité. In: *Le Droit de mentir, B. Constant, E. Kant*, textes présentés par C. Morana, Paris: Fayard, pp. 17–40.

Couch, S.R. and Kroll-Smith, S., 1997. Environmental movements and expert knowledge: Evidence for a new populism. *International Journal of Contemporary Sociology*, 34, pp. 185–210.

Coulter, A, 1999. Paternalism or partnership? *British Medical Journal*, 319, pp. 719–20.

Coulter, A., Enstwistle, V. and Gilbert, D., 1999. Sharing decision with patients: is the information good enough? *British Medical Journal*, 318, pp. 318–22.

Cresson, G., 2000. La confiance dans la relation médecin/patient. In: Cresson G. and Schweyer F.-X. eds., *Les usagers du système de soins*. Rennes: ENSP, pp. 333–50.

Degner, L.F. and Sloan, J.A., 1992. Decision-making during serious illness: what role do patients really want to play? *Journ. Clin. Epidemiol.*, 45(9), pp. 941–50.

Delaporte, C., 2001. *Dire la vérité au malade*. Paris: Odile Jacob.

Delcey, M., 2001. Quelle information pour permettre un exercice effectif des droits des malades? *Actualité et Dossier en Santé Publique*, 36, pp. 56–7.

Demma, F., Douiller, A., Fervers, B., Sandrin-Berthon, B., Saltel, P. and Philip, T., 1999. Les besoins d'information et de communication des personnes atteints de cancer (ce qu'en exprime un groupe de patients). *La santé de l'homme*, 341, pp. 24–7.

Dentan, R.K., 1970. Living and working with the Semai. In: G.D. Spindler ed., *Being an anthropologist: fieldwork in eleven cultures*. New York: Holt, Rinehart & Winston, pp. 85–112.

Dodier, N., 2002. Recomposition de la médecine dans ses rapports avec la science. Les leçons du sida. *Santé publique et sciences sociales*, 8–9, pp. 37–52.

Dozon, J.-P. and Vidal, L. eds., 1993. *Les sciences sociales face au sida*. Paris: Editions de l'Orstom.

Drewermann, E., 1992. *Le mensonge et le suicide*. Paris: Le Cerf.

Dumoulin, J., 1981. *Le secret professionnel et les embarras de la médecine*. Grenoble: Univ. des sciences sociales de Grenoble/IREPD.

Durandin, G., 1972. *Les fondements du mensonge*. Paris: Flammarion.

Durandin, G., 1993. *L'information, la désinformation et la réalité*. Paris: PUF.

Ekman, P., 1985. *Telling lies. Clues to deceit in the marketplace, politics and marriage.* New York/London: W. W. Norton & Cie.

Fainzang, S., 1996. *Ethnologie des anciens alcooliques. La liberté ou la mort.* Paris: Presses Universitaires de France.

Fainzang, S., 2001. *Médicaments et Sociétés. Le patient, le médecin et l'ordonnance.* Paris: Presses Universitaires de France.

Fainzang, S., 2006. Transmission et circulation des savoirs sur les médicaments dans la relation médecin-malade. In: *Le médicament au cœur de la socialité contemporaine. Regards croisés sur un objet complexe.* J. Collin, M. Otero, L. Monnais eds. Québec: Presses de l'Univ. du Québec, pp. 267–79.

Fainzang, S., 2012. *L'automédication ou les mirages de l'autonomie.* Paris: Presses Universitaires de France.

Fan, R., 1997. Self-determination versus family determination: two incommensurable principles of autonomy. *Bioethics*, 11, pp. 309–22.

Favereau, E., 1994. *Le silence des médecins.* Paris: Calmann-Lévy.

Fillion, E., 2003. How is medical decision-making shared? The case of Haemophilia patients and doctors: the aftermath of the infected blood affair in France. *Health Expectations*, 66(3), pp. 228–41.

Fletcher, J., 1979. *Morals and medicine. The moral problems of the patient's right to know the truth.* New Jersey: Princeton University Press.

Foucault, M., 1980. *Power/knowledge, selected interviews and other writings, 1972–1977.* Colin Gordon ed. New York: Pantheon Books.

Frank, A., 1991. *The Will of the Body.* Chicago: University of Chicago Press.

Furst, L.R., 1998. *Between doctors and patients. The changing balance of power.* Charlottesville/London: University Press of Virginia.

Geets, C., 1993. Vérité et mensonge dans la relation au malade. *Revue d'éthique et de théologie morale*, 184, pp. 56–77.

Ghadi, V., 2001. Information des usagers. *Actualité et dossier en santé publique*, 36, pp. 36–9.

Ghadi, V. and Polton, D., 2000. Le marché ou le débat comme instruments de la démocratie. *Revue française des Affaires sociales*, 2, pp. 15–32.

Giddens, A., 1987. *La constitution de la société.* Paris: PUF.

Giddens, A., 1991. *The transformation of intimacy.* Cambridge: Polity Press.

Giddens, A., 1991. *Modernity and self-identity.* Cambridge: Polity Press.

Gillot, D., 2000. Sur la démocratie sanitaire. *Revue française des Affaires sociales*, 2, pp. 5–7.

Gordon, D.R., 1991. Culture, cancer and communication in Italy. In: *Anthropologies of medicine*, B. Pfleiderer and G. Bibeau eds. *Curare*, 7, pp. 137–56.

Grigsby, J. and Sanders, J.H., 1998. Telemedicine: Where it is and where it's going. *Annals of Internal Medicine*, 129, pp. 123–7.

Gruénais, M.E., 1993. Dire ou ne pas dire. Enjeux de l'annonce de la séropositivité à Brazzaville (Congo). In: J.P. Dozon and L. Vidal eds., *Les sciences sociales face au sida. Cas africains autour de l'exemple ivoirien.* Centre Orstom de Petit-Bassam, GIDIS-CI/Orstom, pp. 207–20.

Guillet, P., 2001. Droits des malades, information et responsabilité. Editorial. *ADSP*, 36, p. 1.

Hacking, I., 1982. Language, truth and reason. In: Hollis M. and Lukes S. eds., *Rationality and relativism.* Oxford: Basil Blackwell, pp. 48–66.

Hardey, M., 1999. Doctor in the house. *Sociology of Health and Illness*, 12(6), pp. 820–35.

Hardey, M., 2001. E-health: The Internet and transformation patients into consumers and the producers of health knowledge. *Information, Communication and Society*, 4(1), pp. 388–405.

Hardey, M., 2004. Internet et société: reconfigurations du patient et de la médecine? *Sciences sociales et santé*, 22(1), pp. 5–20.

Henderson, L.J., 1970 (1935). Physician and patient as a social system. In: *On the social system: selected writing.* Chicago: University of Chicago Press, pp. 202–13.

Higgins, R.W., 1986. Aspects philosophiques de la vérité. *Jalmav*, 7, pp. 5–10.

Hippocrate, 1994. *De l'art médical.* Paris: Le Livre de poche.

Hirsh, E., 1999. *La relation médecin/malade face aux exigences de l'information.* Paris: AP-HP/Doin.

Hoerni, B., 1985. *Paroles et silences du médecin.* Paris: Flammarion.

Hoerni, B., 1991. *Nouvelles relations entre les personnes malades et les personnes soignantes.* Paris: Payot, Bibliothèque scientifique.

Hoerni, B., 1999. Communiquer l'information médicale. De nouvelles responsabilités partagées. In: Hirsch E. ed. *La relation médecin-malade face aux exigences de l'information.* Paris: AP-HP/ Doin, pp. 37–40.

Hoerni, B., 1999. Principes et pratiques d'un secret: le secret médical. In: Frison-Roche M.-A. ed., *Secrets professionnels.* Paris: Editions Autrement, Essais, pp. 177–89.

Hoerni, B., 2005. Vie et déclin du 'mensonge médical'. *Histoire des sciences médicales*, 39(4), pp. 349–58.

Hoerni, B. and Soubeyran, P., 2004. Histoire de l'information aux personnes atteintes de cancer. *Cancers et société*, 21, pp. 13–38.

Hogg, C., 1999. *Patients, power and politics. From patients to citizens.* London: Sage Publications.

Holland, J.C., Geary, N., Marchini, A. and Tross, S., 1987. An international survey of physician attitudes and practice in regard to revealing the diagnosis of cancer. *Cancer Investigation*, 5(2), pp. 151–4.

Hooper, E.M., Comstock, L.M., Goodwin, J.M. and Goodwin, J.S., 1982. Patient characteristics that influence physician behavior. *Medical Care*, 20(6), pp. 630–38.

Israël, L., 1992. *Vivre avec un cancer.* Paris: Editions du Rocher.

Jaffré, Y., 2002. Trop proche ou trop lointain. La construction de la relation entre soignants et soignés dans un service d'hémato-oncologie au Mali. *Santé publique et sciences sociales*, 8–9, pp. 119–44.

Jamin, J., 1977. *Les lois du silence. Essai sur la fonction sociale du secret*. Paris: Maspéro.

Jamous, R., 1993. Mensonge, violence et silence dans le monde méditerranéen. *Terrain*, 21, pp. 97–110.

Jobert, B., 2000. Les institutions sanitaires à l'épreuve. Quatre dimensions de l'action démocratique. *Revue française des Affaires sociales*, 2, pp. 33–43.

Joseph-Jeanneney, B., Bréchot, J.M. and Ruszniewski, M., 2002. *Autour du malade. La famille, le médecin et le psychologue*. Paris: Odile Jacob.

Journal officiel, 2002. *Les relations entre médecins et patients. Les principaux textes de loi*. Paris: Direction des Journaux officiels.

Katz, J., 1984. *The silent world of doctor and patient*. NY/London: The Free Press.

Khodoss, H., 2000. Démocratie sanitaire et droits des usagers. *Revue française des Affaires sociales*, 2, pp. 111–22.

Konior, G.S. and Levine, A.S., 1975. The fear of dying: how patients and their doctors behave. *Semin Oncol*, 2, pp. 311–16.

Koyré, A., 1996 (1944). *Réflexions sur le mensonge*. Paris: Editions Allia.

Koyré, A., 1947. *Epiménide le menteur. Ensemble et catégorie*. Paris: Hermann.

Kuran, T., 1995. *Private truths, public lies. The social consequences of preference falsification*. Cambridge (Mass)/London: Harvard University Press.

Lagrée, J., 2002. *Le médecin, le malade et le philosophe*. Paris: Bayard.

Lahoute, C., 2000. Droit des usagers du système de santé. De la réglementation à la pratique. In: Cresson G. and Schweyer F.X. eds., *Les usagers du système de soins*. Rennes, Editions de l'Ecole Nationale de Santé Publique, pp. 17–24.

La Revue Agora, 1996. Le secret. 37.

Lascoumes P., 2002. Représenter les usagers. In: I. Baszanger, M. Bungener and A. Paillet eds., *Quelle médecine voulons-nous?* Paris: La Dispute, pp. 107–25.

Letourmy, A. and Naiditch, M., 2000. L'information des usagers sur le système de soins : rhétorique et enjeux. *Revue française des Affaires sociales*, 2, pp. 45–60.

Levy-Soussan, M., 2004. Subjectivité du malade et normes médicales, Séminaire du SIRS: *Représentations de santé et construction des normes* Available at: http://www.u707.jussieu.fr/sirs/Rencontre%204%20Novembre%202004.doc [accessed 12 January 2005].

Ligue nationale contre le cancer, 1999. *Les malades prennent la parole. Le livre blanc des 1ers Etats généraux des malades du cancer*. Paris: Ramsay.

Louis-Courvoisier, M., 2001. Le malade et son médecin: le cadre de la relation thérapeutique dans la 2ème moitié du 18ème siècle. *Bulletin canadien d'histoire de la médecine*, 18, pp. 277–96.

MacIntosh, J., 1976. Patients' awareness and desire for information about diagnosed but undisclosed malignant disease. *Lancet*, 2, pp. 300–303.

Macklin, R., 1999. *Against relativism. Cultural diversity and the search for ethical universals in medicine*. New York/Oxford: Oxford University Press.

Maheu, E., 1996. Secret et transparence: un enjeu démocratique. *La Revue Agora*, 37, pp. 3–8.

Massé, R., 2003. *Ethique et santé publique, Enjeux, valeurs et normativité*. Québec: Presses de l'Université de Laval.

Massé, R. and Légaré, F., 2001. The limitations of a negociation model for perimenopausal women. *Sociology of Health & Medicine*, 23(1), pp. 44–64.

Meichenbaum, D, and Turk, D.C., 1987. *Facilitating treatment adherence: A practitioner's guidebook*. New York/London: Plenum Press.

Ménoret, M., 1999. *Les temps du cancer*. Paris: Editions du CNRS.

Mintzes, B., 2001. Doctor, about that medicine I saw advertised …, Available at: http://www.inmotionmagazine.com/hcare/mintzes.html [accessed 14 June 2004].

Moley-Massol, I., 2004. *L'annonce de la maladie. Une parole qui engage*. Courbevoie: DaTebe Editions (Coll. La Pratique).

Morana, C. (textes présentés par), 2003. *Le Droit de mentir, B. Constant, E. Kant*. Paris: Fayard.

Moumjid-Ferdjaoui, N. and Carrère, M.O., 2000. La relation médecin-patient, l'information et la participation des patients à la décision médicale: les enseignements de la littérature internationale. *Revue française des Affaires sociales*, 2, pp. 73–88.

Nyberg, D., 1993. *The varnished truth. Truth telling and deceiving in ordinary life*. Chicago: University of Chicago Press.

Oken, D., 1961. What to tell cancer patients. A study of medical attitudes. *JAMA*, 175, pp. 1120–28.

Olender, M., 1983. D'un préjugé que certains nomment vérité. *Le Genre humain*, 7–8, pp. 7–9.

Ong, L.M.L., de Haes, J.C., Hoos, A.M. and Lammes, F.B., 1995. Doctor/patient communication: a review of the literature. *Social Science & Medicine*, 40(7), pp. 903–18.

Perez, Z., 1996. The Historical Significance of Lying and Dissimilation. *Social Research*, 63, pp. 863–912.

Perpère, A., 2004. Impact de l'accès à Internet dans la relation médecin/malade en cancérologie. Réflexions à partir d'un cas clinique. *Revue francophone de psycho-oncologie*, 4, pp. 216–22.

Petitat, A., 1998. *Secret et formes sociales*. Paris: PUF.

Pierret, J., 1998. La question de l'acceptabilité et de l'information. In: *Risques héréditaires de cancers du sein et de l'ovaire. Quelle prise en charge?* Paris: Editions de l'INSERM (Coll. Expertise collective), pp. 281–92.

Platon, 1966. *La République*. Paris: Garnier-Flammarion.

Ponchon, F., 1998. *Le secret professionnel à l'hôpital et l'information du malade*. Paris: Berger-Levrault.

Rabaté, J.-M., 2005. *Tout dire ou ne rien dire. Logiques du mensonge*. Paris: Stock.

Rabeharisoa, V. and Callon, M., 1999. *Le pouvoir des malades. L'Association française contre les myopathies et la Recherche*. Paris: Presses de l'Ecole des mines.

Radstake, M., 2000. *Secrecy and ambiguity. Home care for people living with HIV/AIDS in Ghana*, African Studies Centre, Research Report 59, Leiden.

Rameix, S., 1997. Du paternalisme des soignants à l'autonomie des patients? *Laennec*, 1, pp. 10–15.

Reich, M., 2004. L'information diagnostique et pronostique à l'épreuve des avancées thérapeutiques en cancérologie: réflexions éthiques. *Revue Psycho-oncologie*, 3(4), pp. 188–96.

René, L. 1996. Le secret médical: vertu bourgeoise ou valeur humaniste. *La Revue Agora*, 37, pp. 109–14.

Revue française des Affaires sociales, 2000. La démocratie sanitaire, 54, 2.

Revue Prescrire, 1999. Visite médicale: le bilan accablant du Réseau d'observation de la revue Prescrire, 19(193), pp. 226–31.

Roqueplo, P., 1974. *Le partage du savoir*. Paris: Le Seuil.

Rosman, S., 2003. Cancer and stigma: experience of patients with chemotherapy-induced alopecia. *Patient Education & Counseling*, 52, pp. 333–9.

Ruszniewski, M., 1995. *Face à la maladie grave. Patients, familles, soignants*. Paris: Privat/Dunot.

Saillant, F., 1988. *Cancer et Culture. Produire le sens de la maladie*. Montréal: Editions Saint-Martin.

Santé conjuguée, 2005. La communication et l'information en santé, 33, pp. 23–119.

Sarradon-Eck, A., Vega, A., Faure, M., Humbert-Gaudart, A. and Lustman, M., 2004. *Etude qualitative des interactions professionnelles dans les réseaux de soins informels*. Rapport pour l'ANAES.

Schein, E.H., 2004. Learning when and how to lie: a neglected aspect of organizational and occupational socialization. *Human Relations*, 57(3), pp. 260–73.

Schnitzler, A., 2002. *Mourir*. Paris: Stock.

Shibles, W., 1985. *Lying: A critical analysis*. Whitewater, Wisconsin: The Language Press.

Sicard, D., 2000. Le médecin et ses malades – le malade et ses médecins. In: Y. Michaud, ed. *Qu'est-ce que l'humain?* 2, *Université de tous les savoirs*. Paris: Odile Jacob, pp. 551–8.

Simmel, G., 1991. *Secret et sociétés secrètes*. Translated from German by S. Muller. Strasbourg: Circé.

Strauss, A.L. and Baszanger, I. (présenté par), 1992. *La trame de la négociation: sociologie qualitative et interactionnisme*. Paris: L'Harmattan.

Street, R.L., 1992. Communicative styles and adaptations in physician-parent consultations. *Social Science & Medicine*, 34(10), pp. 1155–63.

Tambiah, S.J., 1990. *Magic, science, religion and the scope of rationality*. Cambridge/ New York: Cambridge University Press.

Thouvenin, D., 2000. Rapports entre patients, soignants et institutions; les enjeux d'une évolution. *Revue française des Affaires sociales*, 2, pp. 33–5.

Van Dongen, E. and Fainzang, S. eds., 2005. *Lying and illness. Power and performance*. Amsterdam: Het Spinhuis.

Vennin, P., Hecquet, B., Marcuzzi, I. and Demaille, M.C., 1995. Cancer du sein. L'information en question(s). Enquête auprès des patientes et des médecins d'un centre de lutte contre le cancer. *Bulletin du Cancer*, 82, pp. 698–704.

Vial, A., 1999. Information e(s)t promotion. *Actualité et Document en santé publique*, 27, pp. 65–7.

Walton, D., 1995. *A pragmatic theory of fallacy*. Tuscaloosa/London: The University of Alabama Press.

Wise, D., 1973. *The politics of lying: Government deception, secrecy and power*. New York: Random House.

Wyatt, S., Henvood, F., Hart, A. and Platzer, H., 2004. L'extension des territoires du patient: Internet et santé au quotidien. *Sciences sociales et santé*, 22(1), pp. 45–68.

Zempléni, A., 1976. La chaîne du secret. *Nouvelle revue de psychanalyse*, 14, pp. 313–24.

Index

and medical nomadism 100–101
by patients 97–104
by omission 101–2
and power 55, 136
prevalence of 49
and social order, maintenance of
53–4
as social phenomenon 1
and things left unsaid 52–3
see also secrets; truth

Macklin, R. 92
Massé, R. 33
mastectomy 44, 64, 126
medical files, patients' access to 6,
86fn6
Ménoret, Marie 71
Merran, S. 52
metastases
disclosure of 37–8, 52, 91, 98,
115, 117
lung 120
misunderstandings
cognitive discrepancy 124–5, 134
examples 111–19
and insufficient medical
information 125
knowledge 126–7
and medical jargon 119–24, 131,
135
and unanswered questions 127–9

Nuremberg Code 8
nurses, as doctors' spokespersons
47–8

oedema, brain 122
oncologists 21, 29, 33, 36
status 70
Ong, L.M.L 76

pain 72, 80, 96, 99, 102
doctors' disregard of 81
inappropriate treatment 87

palliative care 11, 25, 57, 73, 89, 108,
120
Parsons, T. 86
patient associations 3, 4, 6, 7, 12, 28,
37, 38, 96
patients
autonomy 92
diagnosis
prior knowledge of 87–8
requests to withhold from
90–91
entourage 90–91
lying *see* lying, by patients
minimising of symptoms 77–8
rights 6
see also information, and patients
Patients' Rights Act (2002) 9, 36
Plato, *Republic* 52
pneumococcus 100
Ponchon, F. 7
power
and lying 55, 136
and secrets 56, 57
prognosis
and diagnosis 23, 37–8, 91
patients' refusal to accept 89
Promotion of Patients' in Europe,
Declaration 6, 9
psychologists
distrust of 16
on doctors 31, 49, 50
role 48–9
Public Health Code 5, 8
Pujol, Henri 28

radiologists 46
radiotherapy 78, 114
research project
demographic profile 11
diseases studied 10
interviews 12–13
methodology 11–12
number of patients 10
observer's behaviour 13–18